THE ACUPUNCTURE TREATMENT OF INTERNAL DISEASE

An introduction to the use of traditional Chinese acupuncture in the treatment
of some common internal diseases

by

George T. Lewith
M.A., M.R.C.G.P., M.R.C.P.

Illustrated by Stephen Lee

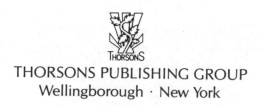

THORSONS PUBLISHING GROUP
Wellingborough · New York

First published 1985

British Library Cataloguing in Publication Data

Lewith, G. T.
   The acupuncture treatment of internal disease:
   an introduction to the use of traditional
   Chinese acupuncture in the treatment of some
   common internal diseases
   1. Acupuncture
   I. Title
   615.8'92   RM184

   ISBN 0-7225-1103-5

Printed and bound in Great Britain.

Contents

Preface

This book provides a concise introduction to the use of traditional Chinese medicine in the treatment of some common internal diseases. The diseases are given a Western diagnosis and then the appropriate and common organ dysfunctions that lead to that diagnostic category are discussed. In the classical traditional sense where diagnoses are made by using the twelve pulses, almost any organ can be affected in almost any condition. However, in order to provide a practical introduction to the treatment of these conditions it is much easier to work on the basis of the practitioner's current knowledge. The system of differentiation of syndromes within the limit of an allopathic diagnosis, is the current approach used in China to treat internal problems.

My aim in writing this book is to take the treatment of such problems away from the realms of a simple point prescription, but not to suggest that point selection is so complex that it makes it almost impossible for the acupuncturist to know where to start. However tortuous the paradigms and systems of traditional Chinese medicine may at first seem, they do provide a framework within which the acupuncturist can work in order to choose the most appropriate points for specific problems.

The book describes the general principles of treatment for approximately forty common internal diseases. Its aim is to guide the aspiring acupuncturist towards treatment and management in conditions other than pain, where a simple, safe technique such as acupuncture can certainly be of value.

It has been difficult enough to 'prove' the effects of acupuncture as an analgesic. Modern scientific methods of testing treatment efficacy (double blind controlled trials) do not readily lend themselves to physical therapies such as acupuncture. However, the evidence available does suggest that acupuncture is definitely a useful and powerful analgesic therapy. Its place in the treatment of many internal diseases, particularly with respect to the comparison of acupuncture with allopathic therapy, is unclear. Consequently I do not wish to imply that acupuncture is the best treatment for the conditions discussed; considerably more comparative research is required before a rank order of treatments can be defined. Nevertheless acupuncture does appear to have a value (both from my own experience and that of the Chinese) in the conditions mentioned.

G. T. LEWITH
Southampton, 1985

Introduction

The neurophysiological mechanisms initiated by acupuncture, or needle puncture, have been clearly documented with respect to the effect of acupuncture as an analgesic therapy. It is now well known and widely accepted that acupuncture affects neural transmission both peripherally and centrally, and that it promotes the release of a variety of endogenous opiates which can in some instances be shown to relieve pain. However, the effects of acupuncture on painful conditions do not provide explanations as to how acupuncture may be working in diseases such as cerebrovascular accidents or colitis.

Acupuncture has been used as a therapy for many non-painful conditions, and a clear effect from acupuncture has been reported on the immune system, [1,2] the gall bladder [3] and the coronary arteries. [4] Acupuncture has also been shown to cause a number of fundamental changes in the autonomic system [5] and several experiments attest to its influence on the gastro-intestinal tract. [6,7,8] These studies demonstrate that acupuncture is having a very fundamental effect on aspects of the nervous system that control internal functions rather than just pain and they represent only a small part of a growing body of literature that describes the actions of acupuncture in non-painful conditions.

These changes have been poorly studied by Western researchers; furthermore very few clinical trials have been published which have attempted to evaluate the symptomatic or curative effects of acupuncture on non-painful conditions. Consequently we know very little about the mechanism and the clinical effects of acupuncture in such situations. In the early 1960s acupuncture was thought of as no more than quackery, it was almost beyond the imagination that such clear physiological evidence for its analgesic properties would emerge. Perhaps this story may be repeated with respect to the treatment of internal disease, when resources are made available to investigate the many claims for its effects in non-painful conditions.

PART ONE: THE TREATMENT

1.

Traditional Chinese Medicine

The theory of yin and yang is a kind of world outlook. It holds that all things have two opposite aspects, yin and yang, which are interdependent while at the same time being at two extremes. The Chinese believe this to be a universal law of the material world. Yin and yang are interdependent because one cannot exist without the presence of the other. The ancient Chinese used water and fire to symbolize yin and yang; anything moving, hot, bright, hyperactive or non-substantive was considered to be yang, while anything quiescent, cold, dim, hypoactive or substantive was considered to be yin.

The yin and yang properties of things are not absolute but relative. As an object or person changes, so the yin and yang components change at a gradual rate. Each of the positive or negative properties of an object is a condition for the existence of its opposite; neither can exist in isolation. These two opposites are not stationary but in constant motion. If we imagine the circadian rhythm, night is yin and day is yang; as night (yin) fades, it becomes day (yang), and as yang fades, it becomes yin. Yin and yang are therefore changing into each other as well as balancing each other.

At first these philosophical ideas may seem very simplistic, but on closer analysis such an approach represents a series of very profound concepts. Each organ has an element of yin, and yang, within it, the structures and nutrients tend to be designated as yin and the functional activities as yang. Some organs are mainly yang in nature (functional) such as the gan-liver, while others are mainly yin (structural) such as the shen-kidney. Even though one organ may be more yin in nature, that organ will also have yang properties. Furthermore, the balance of yin and yang is maintained in the healthy body because the sum total of yin and yang will be in fluctuant balance. Western medicine is very good at defining disease, but is presented with almost insurmountable difficulties when attempting to define health. The assumptions within traditional Chinese medicine imply that health is an almost unattainable ideal, because yin and yang are always fluctuating and never quite completely balanced. This means that one day you feel well while another you don't feel quite up to par. For most of us this represents a fairly normal existence, what we would usually call good health. Disease is looked upon as a process where yin and yang are in permanent imbalance. Either yin or yang may be in excess or deficiency. A disease in which the primary event is an *excess* of either yin or yang is called a *shi disease*. Most shi diseases are acute conditions, for instance tonsillitis represents invasion by the pathogen heat, is an acute disease, and also one of excess (shi). A *xu disease* is one of *deficiency*, for instance arthritis in an old person almost always occurs because the substance (yin) of their shen-kidney begins to wear out (as we will see later, the shen-kidney dominates bone). Consequently most chronic diseases are considered xu.

Channels and Collaterals

These are representations of the organs of the body, in a functional rather than a material sense. Qi, or vital energy, flows through the channels, and if the organ which the channel represents is malfunctioning then the Chinese believe the flow of qi through that channel is disturbed. This assumption, while attractive, is currently impossible to validate within the paradigms of conventional science.

The essential principle of acupuncture is to use points on the channels to correct the flow of qi through the channels, thereby returning the organ to its normal function and restoring the normal yin/yang balance within the body. The exact location of the twelve meridians and methods of point location and measurement will be dealt with in a later chapter.

Qi

Qi is a complex concept, it relates both to substance and function. Clean qi (oxygen), waste qi (carbon dioxide) and qi (nutrients) are generally known as material qi. The existence of material qi is shown by the functional activity of an organ, the qi of that organ. A dead organ has no functional activity and therefore no qi. Therefore qi or vital energy is considered as both substantive (material) and functional (non-material). It is a concept that is difficult to understand and at times seems all-embracing, but nevertheless it is of value when attempting to understand the paradigms of traditional Chinese medicine.

The Zang and Fu Organs

In very simple terms zang means solid organs and fu means hollow organs, although the heart in real terms is a hollow organ, but nevertheless is considered to be zang. The zang organs are the liver, kidney, heart, lung, spleen and pericardium (sometimes called the circulation in some Western texts). Throughout this book they will be referred to as the gan-liver, shen-kidney, xin-heart, fei-lung and pi-spleen. This is not just aimed at exercising the reader's skill in Mandarin pronunciation, but is a deliberate effort to continually remind the reader that while the gan-liver has many similar functions to that of the liver within conventional medicine, some of the functions within traditional Chinese medicine are different but equally important. Therefore prefixing the liver with its Mandarin name, gan, will continually remind the reader of both aspects of the liver's function.

The zang organs are more important than the fu organs in that most diseases result from either internal dysfunction, or invasion by a pathogen causing dysfunction, of a zang organ. On the whole, the fu organs have similar functions to those in Western medicine and are less likely to be the major cause of a disease.

The Zang Organs

1. *The gan-liver*

   This is the main yang organ of the body. It takes charge of the free flow of blood and qi through all the tissues and channels of the body. It controls muscle tone and has its orifice through the eye. Symptoms of spasm or spasticity as well as pain or disease referred to the eye are likely to be due to dysfunction of the gan-liver. The gan-liver is linked both structurally and functionally to the gall-bladder channel.

2. *The shen-kidney*

   This is the main yin organ of the body. It dominates growth, reproduction and bone metabolism, as well as controlling the acid base balance and body fluid in conjunction with the fei-lung. The shen-kidney has the ear as its orifice, consequently symptoms referred to the ear such as tinnitus may be treated by using points on the kidney channel. The shen-kidney is linked structurally and functionally to the urinary bladder.

3. *The xin-heart*

   The xin-heart dominates the circulation of blood. However, its main function seems to be the maintenance of normal mentality, the Chinese refer to this function as, 'keeping the mind'. The xin-heart has its orifice through the tongue and is linked structurally and functionally to the small intestine channel.

4. *The fei-lung*

   The fei-lung necessarily controls respiration, but also dominates hair and skin. It has a major influence on water metabolism within the body in conjunction with the shen-kidney and takes the nose as its orifice. Therefore symptoms referred to the upper respiratory tract can be treated by using points on the lung channel. The large intestine channel and lung channel are linked, and points on the large intestine channel are particularly useful in treating diseases of the fei-lung.

5. *The pi-spleen*

   The pi-spleen's main function is digestion, and the transportation and distribution of digestive products throughout the body. In the context of traditional Chinese medicine it takes over the function of the stomach, small intestine and large intestine. As a consequence the pi-spleen dominates the nutritional status of the body, being in control of muscle bulk and general health. It stops extravasation of blood and takes the mouth as its orifice. It is linked both structurally and functionally to the stomach and many stomach points act synergistically with points on the spleen channel.

6. *The pericardium*
   In some Western texts the pericardium is known as the circulation channel. Its functions are really those of the xin-heart, and in functional terms it doesn't really exist in isolation. It has no Chinese prefix.

The Fu Organs

The Fu organs are the small intestine, gall-bladder, stomach, large intestine, urinary bladder and sanjiao. Each of the fu organs is linked both structurally and functionally to a zang organ; these connections have already been stated. The function of the fu organs is almost exactly the same as in allopathic medicine, the only difference being that of the sanjiao.

The sanjiao
In Chinese the sanjiao means three cavities. The xin-heart and the fei-lung are in the upper jiao (the chest), the pi-spleen and stomach are in the middle jiao (the epigastrium) and the shen-kidney and bladder in the lower jiao (the hypogastrium). The sanjiao is sometimes called the *triple warmer* or *triple heater* organ. One of its main functions is said to be controlling the balance of heat between these three body cavities, it's also said to have important endocrine functions and you will note in the diseases that follow that the points on the sanjiao are frequently used.

Pathogens

Pathogenic factors are those which cause disease, they can be divided into two main groups, exogenous pathogens, and internal or mental pathogens. If the body is out of balance, for whatever reason, then its qi and consequently its ability to resist disease is inadequate. Therefore the pathogens or pathogenic qi may invade and cause disease. It is important within the context of traditional Chinese medicine to isolate the disease-causing factor or pathogen so that appropriate therapy can be given to overcome it.

1. *The exogenous pathogens*
   The Chinese classify the exogenous pathogens within a variety of symptom complexes that are typified by meteorological terms.

   Heat. Heat really means if a person is hot or a particular disease presents with the symptoms of heat. For instance tonsillitis would be a disease of heat as it is associated with a systemic fever; an infected joint would be locally hot and is due (within the paradigms of traditional Chinese medicine) to the local invasion of heat. If the heat is mild it may be described as warmth, if it is acute and severe it may be described as fire. Particular acupuncture points are available which can be used to disperse heat. These are: LI4, LI11, Du14.

   Cold. Invasion by cold usually indicates a chronic or xu disease. Osteoarthritis is often a disease of cold in that it is a chronic disease, the symptoms of which often get worse during the autumn and winter. Many chronic diseases treated with acupuncture (particularly chronic arthritis) will have cold as a pathogen. In diseases where local

14

invasion of cold is apparent, for instance in osteoarthritis of the knee, then local heat should be used. If there is systemic invasion of cold, for instance in chronic gastrointestinal problems, the following points may be used to disperse cold systemically: Ren6, Sp10, St36.

These points should be treated by the use of needling and moxibustion.

Wind. Wind is a symptom complex that is changeable. The viral arthritis frequently experienced during an attack of influenza would be typical of the pathogen wind. The specific points to disperse wind are: LI4, LI11.

Damp. Damp is muddy, sticky and greasy. It is a pathogen that commonly invades obese people who have dysfunction of the pi-spleen; damp almost invariably invades via the pi-spleen. It is typified by diseases of indigestion and usually the patient will present with a greasy tongue. The point to disperse damp is St40.

Phlegm. Phlegm is a pathological product. Within the context of traditional Chinese medicine, phlegm is present only when damp invades; phlegm is a secondary product of damp. In many ways the pathogen phlegm is a symptom more substantive in concept than damp.

Point to disperse phlegm is St40.

St40 is often used in combination with Sp6 because phlegm and damp frequently invade through the pi-spleen.

2. *The mental pathogens*

The mental or internal pathogens are *overjoy, anger, anxiety, overthinking, grief, fear and fright.*

Excessive fear, fright or overjoy injure the xin-heart. This results in palpitations, insomnia, irritability, anxiety and other mental abnormalities.

Excessive anger damages the gan-liver. This impairs its function resulting in depression and irritability.

Excessive grief, anxiety and over-thinking cause dysfunction of the pi-spleen; this results in anorexia and a feeling of fullness or distension after meals.

It is interesting to note that the Chinese believe that excessive grief, anxiety and anger cause a poor circulation of qi and blood. This can result in cancer, an observation that has recently been made within the context of Western medicine.

2.

Principles of Therapy

Diseases fall into two main groups; diseases of the channels and collaterals and diseases of the zang and fu organs.

1. Diseases of the Channels and Collaterals

These are diseases of the superficial channels of the body. Arthritis and acute strains are examples of this type of disease. The internal yin/yang balance is normal, but the flow of qi and blood through the channels is disrupted. This usually presents with pain, and is called a disease of 'Bi' or blockage of the channels. If the flow of qi and blood is restored, then the pain will go, and this is the main therapeutic principle for this type of disease.

These diseases can be treated solely on the basis of local points around the site of pain, and distal points on the channel that runs over the pain. The principle of local and distal points is an important one.

The local point is usually quite obvious; it is either felt as a local tender area, or as a small pea-sized nodule under the skin. The distal point is less obvious and has to be learnt. The distal points are:

LI4 — this point may be used for pain over the large intestine channel. It is also a very important point for facial pain, headache and sinusitis.

LI11 — is often used as a distal point for referred pain from the shoulder or neck.

SJ5 — is the most important point on the upper limb. If there is pain on the upper limb, that is not on a channel, then this point may be used. It is also used when there is pain over the sanjiao channel.

UB40 — this point is used for low back pain, or any pain over the lower part of the urinary bladder channel.

UB60 — this point is used for upper thoracic, cervical pain, or headache. It is used for pain over the upper part of the urinary bladder channel.

GB34 — this may be used for pain over the gall-bladder channel, such as migraine.

St44 — this is used for pain over the stomach channel, such as facial pain or hip pain radiating down the front of the leg.

2. Diseases of the Zang and Fu Organs

These are diseases of the internal organs of the body where there is an imbalance of yin and yang within the body. Vertigo, anxiety and asthma are clear examples of this type of disease. To treat these problems, it is essential to make a clear traditional diagnosis, and to know the rules of point selection.

3. Diseases that Combine Zang-Fu and Channel Disorders

A disease of pain such as migraine, may combine these two ideas. Migraine is usually a disorder of the gan-liver, but there is also a disruption of the flow of qi and blood in the channels over the side of the head, resulting in pain. It is therefore important to treat the gan-liver, i.e., Liv3, and also to treat local and distal points around the site of pain. The local points are usually fairly obvious; often GB20 and Taiyang (Extra) are the local points, and the distal point that should be used is GB34.

4. The Tender Point or Ah Shi Point

Tender points are often found in diseases of pain. The acupuncturist can be guided to this point by the patient stating that they feel pain in a particular area, or by his experience, or by detailed examination. These points may usually be felt as pea-sized nodules under the skin. They should always be used in a disease of pain in combination with local and distal acupuncture points.

18

3.

Methods of Diagnosis

As in conventional medicine the history of the illness is the essential starting point for making a diagnosis. If a patient suggests they are breathless, then the first systems requiring detailed examination would be the heart and lungs. Within the systems used in traditional Chinese medicine similar principles can be applied. For instance, if a patient suggests they have pain or problems referred to the eye then the use of points on the liver channel should be considered; if they have symptoms referred to the nose or upper respiratory tract then the points on the lung and large intestine channel may be required. Therefore a knowledge of organ function, combined with a knowledge of the channels and their internal and external relationships, provides the first and often the most essential step in making a diagnosis and selecting appropriate acupuncture points.

Methods of examination normally applied to Western medicine are also essential within the context of traditional Chinese medicine. However there are two extra examination procedures which are of value within traditional Chinese medicine, the tongue and the pulse.

The Tongue

There are two areas to look at on the tongue, one is the tongue proper (the thin red rim of skin that you see around the edge of the tongue) and the other is the tongue coating, a thin layer on top of the majority of the tongue. A normal tongue has a palish red tongue proper with a thin transparent white coating; most healthy children's tongues are normal. Abnormalities may occur in the tongue proper and/or the tongue coating which will provide the practitioner with a considerable amount of information about which acupuncture points to select.

Tongue Proper

a.   A *pale* coloured tongue proper often with tooth marks, indicates insufficiency of qi and blood and may possibly indicate invasion by cold.

b. A *red* tongue proper indicates diseases of heat, particularly if the tip of the tongue is red it indicates an excess of yang of the gan-liver.

c. A *purplish-red* tongue proper occurs in diseases of severe heat such as a septicaemia or a severe exhaustion of the body fluid such as in terminal cancer.

d. A *purplish* tongue proper can be equated with central cyanosis and indicates a disease of the xin-heart.

e. A *large flabby tooth-marked* tongue proper almost invariably indicates a severe deficiency of qi; this can occur with diseases of the pi-spleen (failure to absorb qi) and/or diseases of the shen-kidney (a deficiency of yin).

Tongue Coating

a. A *thick white* coating indicates invasion by cold. A *greasy white* coating indicates invasion by phlegm and damp, often suggestive of diseases of the pi-spleen.

b. The commonest cause of a *yellow* coating is smoking. If the patient is a non-smoker then a yellow coating indicates invasion by the pathogen heat.

c. A *deficiency* in the tongue coating, usually clinically demonstrable as large gaps in the coating of the tongue, particularly at the back of the tongue, indicates disease of the shen-kidney consuming yin or an excess of the yang of the gan-liver which will also consume yin.

The Pulse

In classical Chinese medicine there are six pulses at each wrist. These pulses occupy three positions, about a centimetre or so apart, over the radial artery on each wrist; each position has a deep and superficial pulse making a total of twelve pulses, and representing the twelve main organs of traditional Chinese medicine. The character of the pulse indicates the state of health of each organ and also the balance between each of the organs. Although traditional diagnosis is still used by some in China and has adherents in the West, I feel that pulse diagnosis is a difficult, if not impossible, skill to grasp competently and the more modern Chinese concept of a pulse 'generalization' is significantly easier to teach and much simpler to learn.

In very general terms, pulses may be classified as excessive or deficient. Most people with acute diseases will have an excessive or full pulse and those with chronic diseases will tend to have a deficient or low volume pulse. There are a number of specific pulse types:

a. *Superficial pulse*. This pulse can be almost abolished by pressure and is often seen in the early stages of disease caused by acute infection.

b. A *deep pulse*. This is only felt on deep palpation and is usually seen in severe internal diseases.

c. A *xu pulse*. This is a weak, forceless and very deficient pulse, and is often seen in diseases of the pi-spleen.

d. A *shi pulse*. This pulse is forceful and does not disappear on palpation; it is seen in diseases of excess.

e. *A threadly pulse.* This is best visualized as a thready flow of water through a tube and is often seen in xu diseases; it can be classified as a pulse indicating deficiency.

f. *A bowstring pulse.* This is hard and forceful and gives a sensation of pressing on the string of a bent bow. In young athletic people it can be normal, but it may also be seen in diseases where there is a hyperacativity of the yang of the gan-liver, for instance in migraine.

g. *A gliding pulse.* This is described by the Chinese as being round and forceful like beads rolling on a plate. It is often seen when phlegm and damp invade and is frequently associated with indigestion.

Diagnostic Controversies

Many of the diseases within Western medicine do not fit easily or simply into a traditional Chinese diagnosis. There are therefore two somewhat extreme views which may guide the practitioner to selecting points for particular internal problems. The first is simply to follow a point prescription; this may suggest that approximately fifty or sixty points could be used to treat a specific disease process such as peptic ulcers. The classical Chinese approach provides the converse view and suggests that the only way to treat a peptic ulcer is to make a diagnosis according to the twelve pulses and then select appropriate points to treat the condition, altering the point selection according to the palpitation of the pulses at each consultation.

Presenting an acupuncturist with a selection of sixty points which may or may not be useful in the specific situation is of limited value, and frequently results in therapeutic failure because there is no basis upon which to choose points in a critical and thoughtful manner. On the other hand the use of traditional pulse diagnosis is a difficult technique to grasp; electronic pulsography as discussed by Julian Kenyon (*Modern Techniques of Acupuncture, Volume II,* 1983, Thorsons) presents a clear and seemingly valid argument which suggests that the traditional pulses do exist and can be used therapeutically to the benefit of the patient. However, in order to apply this information in a critical manner the acupuncturist must purchase an expensive piece of machinery.

In the following sections I have taken a number of common diseases with their Western diagnoses. These have then been subdivided into the most frequent traditional Chinese syndromes that will produce a well-known Western disease pattern. For instance, peptic ulcers may be caused by either a malfunction of the pi-spleen, or by a malfunction of the gan-liver. A point prescription will suggest both liver and spleen points, the patient will only respond clinically if the point selection is based on the functional disturbance within the body. If the diagnosis of that functional disturbance is made too complex, as with diagnosing the twelve pulses, then the acupuncturist may have little more to offer in terms of constructive therapy. Therefore I have adopted the compromise which is currently being used in China. This is achieved by taking a Western disease, analysing the most common traditional Chinese organ imbalances that occur within that disease complex, and suggesting the points (and the reason for the use of each individual point) that would be most appropriate for a particular disease or a particular syndrome that might cause that disease.

The most important aspect of making this modified traditional Chinese diagnosis is to differentiate between the disorders of the five main zang organs. This can be achieved by obtaining information from the history, the pulse and the tongue. The simplified 'sketch' of the zang organs should provide a simple and quick reference in order to differentiate between them. In general the acupuncture point given in the diagram will be enough to correct imbalances within that organ, although a more exacting point selection can be achieved by using the law of the five elements.

Conclusion

Acupuncture can be used to treat pain by the simple expedient of placing needles into the painful areas. Many chronic internal diseases do not present with pain and therefore this very simple approach cannot be used to manage problems such as asthma. Consequently the acupuncturist must make some attempt at making an internal diagnosis using the paradigms of traditional Chinese medicine. The system that I have suggested, while it may have disadvantages when compared with accurate pulse diagnosis, is certainly better than random needle insertion or blind adherence to an ill-understood point prescription.

Organ	Pathogen	Tongue Proper	Tongue Coating	Pulse	Point
Gan-liver	Deficiency of Yin Anger Fire	Red	Yellow or white	Bowstring	Liv3
Shen-kidney	Long excess of Yang Cold	Pale (Tongue can look pale red all over, due to decreased coating)	White Decreased	Xu	K3
Pi-spleen	Damp Phlegm Cold	Pale	White and greasy	Xu or thready	Sp6
Xin-heart	Overjoy Anxiety	Blue	No characteristic tongue coating	Gliding	H7
Fei-lung	Heat Cold	No characteristic tongue coating	Yellow in Heat White in Cold	Gliding and Thready	Lu7

4.

Treatment

When a needle is inserted the acupuncturist must be aware of the underlying tissues and organs. When needling points that are over the lung, needles must be inserted obliquely to avoid the danger of pneumothorax. Commonsense and a knowledge of basic anatomy should avoid any untoward accidents. Needles must also be sterilized properly so that there is no possibility of transmitting serum hepatitis.

It is important to remember that the piece of skin into which you insert the needle is relatively unimportant as long as the needle stimulates the acupuncture point. For instance H7 can be inserted in several different ways, but the acupuncture point has only been stimulated if needling sensation (deqi) is felt. The actual acupuncture point is always underneath the skin and may be an inch or more deep to the dermis. The only way of knowing that you have stimulated an acupuncture point is by obtaining deqi over that point. This means that the tip of the needle is the best point locator that the acupuncturist has at his disposal.

Depth of Needle Insertion
There are only a few simple principles that need to be followed with respect to the choice of the length of needle and actual needle insertion. If needling over a bony area, particularly the scalp, a one-inch needle should be used and inserted obliquely. The same applies to an area where needles are being inserted into thin layers of tissues such as over the face. A one-inch needle should also be used over the distal parts of the body such as the wrist and ankle joint and the hands and feet. If the acupuncturist is going to select points over large joints or muscles such as in the thigh or lower leg then one and a half inch needles should be used and inserted at right angles to the skin. In a well-covered person a two-inch needle may be required. Three-inch needles are required almost exclusively for needling over the buttock, particularly GB30.

Needle Stimulation

Needling sensation or deqi is the most important part of stimulating by needle. This is obtained by manually rotating the needle and, if necessary, at the same time providing a short lifting and thrusting motion. When deqi has been obtained the needling site begins to feel numb and/or dull. Over the scalp, needling sensation may be perceived as a dull burning feeling and occasionally needling sensation may be propagated up and/or down the channels. The easiest test as to whether needling sensation has been achieved is to ask the patient whether the acupuncture needle still feels sharp and like a needle. If the patient reports they still feel a needle is in situ then needling sensation has not been obtained.

Electro-acupuncture or electrical stimulation is required primarily for anaesthesia and the treatment of addictions; the only use that this technique has in the treatment of internal disease is in the management of peripheral nerve injury or cerebrovascular accidents.

Moxibustion and Cupping

In many of the diseases discussed in the following section, *cold* is the important invading *pathogen*. In such situations heat must be applied in order to disperse this pathogen. There are two ways of applying heat, cupping and moxibustion.

1.   *Cupping*

Cupping involves the placing of partially evacuated glass or bamboo cups on the skin. These can be used over the back shu points, and are particularly valuable in the treatment of respiratory diseases such as asthma and bronchitis. It is obviously both impractical and impossible to use cupping on a knee joint or for neck pain, therefore its use is circumscribed to the treatment of points on the thorax, abdomen and back. The cup is placed on the skin by using a lighted flame to produce a partial vacuum and then applying an adroit flick of the hand in order not to dissipate the vacuum created.

2.   *Moxibustion*

Moxibustion involves the use of burning the dried leaves of *Artemesia vulgaris* over or on a point, in order to provide local heat into that point. Moxa may be applied in several different ways:

a)   Loose moxa may be rolled into a cone and burnt directly on the skin. As soon as the cone is partially burnt the patient begins to feel heat; the moxa should be removed at this juncture to avoid scarring. Several moxa cones should be used until a raised reddened area is present over the point that requires heat.

b)   A moxa cone can be burnt on ginger or garlic. The use of ginger or garlic provides some degree of insulation from the direct heat effect of the moxa cone; this method is frequently used on the face, particularly for facial paralysis.

c)   'Warm needling' is used for painful chronic osteoarthritic conditions such as a painful shoulder or cervical osteoarthriosis. An acupuncture needle is inserted, deqi obtained, and then a small section of a moxa stick is placed on the end of the acupuncture needle. The moxa is lighted and heat is conducted by the needle into the deep tissues.

d) Moxa sticks can be lighted, and the lighted end used to heat specific acupuncture points. The moxa stick should not be placed directly on the skin but should be brought up to the skin about a centimetre or so away. This should be repeated on a number of occasions until the area of skin requiring heat is comfortably warm.

e) The Chinese frequently use a moxa box. This is a small wooden box with a zinc grill. Loose moxa is placed into the box and ignited so that diffuse heat can be provided over a circumscribed area of skin. This method is frequently used in the treatment of abdominal conditions, the moxa box being placed over the abdomen in diseases where cold is the invading pathogen.

5.

Guidelines for Treatment

Many Chinese texts suggest that acupuncture treatment should be provided in a series of courses, each course usually involving about eight treatments, and the treatment itself being provided on a daily basis. This almost certainly represents over-treatment and is unnecessary. It is usually quite adequate to provide treatment once a week. At the beginning of treatment it may be necessary to give two or three treatments during the first week or two, and towards the end of treatment therapy may be provided once every two or three weeks. It is important to adjust the treatment frequency in order to balance it against the periodicity of symptoms. If a patient has migraine every month then it is useless to provide half a dozen treatments in the first month without having some assessment as to whether the therapy is being effective; in this instance it would be sensible to plan treatments once every two weeks so that adjustments in point selection can be made if therapy proves to be ineffective in the first instance.

Some of the internal diseases discussed, particularly problems such as cerebrovascular accidents, may require a considerable amount of treatment before some evaluation can be made as to whether therapy is being effective. In some instances the natural history of the disease and response to treatment may become muddled and so occasionally it can be difficult for the acupuncturist to be certain whether the problem is improving spontaneously or whether the therapy is responsible for that improvement. Providing this is explained clearly to the patient and no irresponsible suggestions are made about the effect of acupuncture, it is both logical and ethical to continue with therapy providing the patient continues to improve. In general terms, if there has been no improvement in the patient's condition within four to six treatments, it's unlikely that that condition will improve with the application of acupuncture.

Occasionally reactions to treatment occur; this may involve a slight worsening of the symptoms. It's usually transitory and indicates a response to acupuncture. If a reaction occurs then fewer acupuncture points should be selected on subsequent visits and the needles should be left in for a shorter period of time. The normal duration of treatment is between ten and fifteen minutes. Needling sensation should be obtained on needle insertion and at least once during therapy; for acute (shi) diseases needling sensation should be obtained on a number of occasions during the treatment. For chronic (xu) diseases needling sensation should be obtained only once or perhaps twice during each treatment.

The Channels
There are twelve main channels that run over the body's surface (lung, large intestine, stomach, spleen, heart, small intestine, urinary bladder, kidney, pericardium, sanjiao, gallbladder and liver). In some Western sources the pericardium channel is called the circulation channel, and the sanjiao channel the triple warmer or triple heater. There are two extra channels of importance: the Ren and Du channel. In some Western sources the Ren channel is called the conception channel and the Du the governor channel. *Throughout the text a Chinese numbering system has been applied, as designated by the* Essentials of Chinese Acupuncture, *published by the Foreign Language Press, Peking.*

The Course of the Channels
The course and direction of flow of the qi in the channels is clearly shown in the appended diagrams.

The course of each channel is as follows:

The lung channel begins on the anterior chest wall between the first and second rib. It then passes down the antero-medial aspect of the arm to the medial part of the thumb.

The large intestine channel starts at the nail of the first finger and passes up the antero-lateral aspect of the arm over the shoulder to the face, terminating at the side of the nostril.

The stomach channel starts just below the eye, and then does a 'U' bend over the face passing down through the throat, over the thorax and abdomen down through the front of the thigh and into the foot; it passes between the second and third toes and terminates at the root of the second toe nail.

The spleen channel starts on the big toe, it then travels up the medial aspect of the leg and thigh, over the genitalia, abdomen and thorax. After coming up to the first intercostal space, it terminates in the sixth intercostal space, in a line directly below the axilla.

The heart channel originates in the axilla and runs down the postero-medial aspect of the arm ending at the little finger nail.

The small intestine channel starts at the root of the little finger nail and travels up the postero-lateral aspect of the arm over the scapula and upper thoracic region ending just in front of the ear.

The urinary bladder channel starts on the medial aspect of the orbital cavity, passes over

28

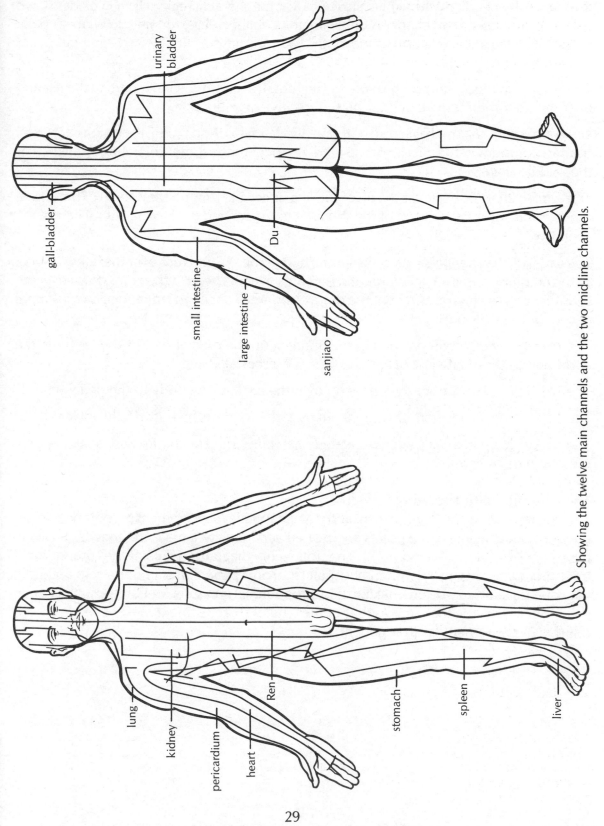

urinary bladder

gall-bladder

small intestine

large intestine

sanjiao

Du

lung

kidney

pericardium

heart

Ren

stomach

spleen

liver

Showing the twelve main channels and the two mid-line channels.

29

the top of the head and then splits into two over the thoracic region. It then passes down the spine and leg as two channels, rejoining the cubital crease, running down the middle of the lower leg and the lateral aspect of the foot, terminating finally on the lateral aspect of the little toe.

The *kidney channel* starts on the sole of the foot, travels up the inner part of the leg and over the abdomen terminating at the sterno-clavicular junction.

The *pericardium channel* begins on the thorax, just lateral to the nipple in the fourth intercostal space. It runs down the middle of the medial aspect of the arm terminating at the nail of the middle finger.

The *sanjiao channel* begins at the tip of the ring finger and runs up the middle of the lateral aspect of the arm, over the tip of the shoulder to the ear and then to the lateral part of the eyebrow.

The *gall-bladder channel* starts at the lateral part of the eye and runs over the lateral aspect of the cranium, passing backwards and forwards over the head. It then runs down over the shoulder and the lateral aspect of the thorax, abdomen and leg, terminating on the lateral aspect of the fourth toe.

The *liver channel* begins on the big toe, running up the medial part of the leg, over the abdomen to terminate just below the fourth intercostal space.

The *Du channel* runs from the upper lip over the back of the body to the perineum.

The *Ren channel* runs from the perineum over the front of the body to the lower lip.

The twelve main channels are represented bilaterally. The Du and Ren channels are only present in the mid-line.

The Cun and Point Location
The cun represents the Chinese inch, and is an adaptable measurement proportional to the patient's build. Many of the points are located according to a measurement of cun away from a clear surface landmark. The following diagrams explain the proportional measurements of the cun (sometimes spelt tsun) on a patient. It is important to ascertain the *patient's* hand size before making these proportional measurements; the examiner's cun will probably not be the same as that of the patient so adjustment *must* be made for the relative measurement for that patient.

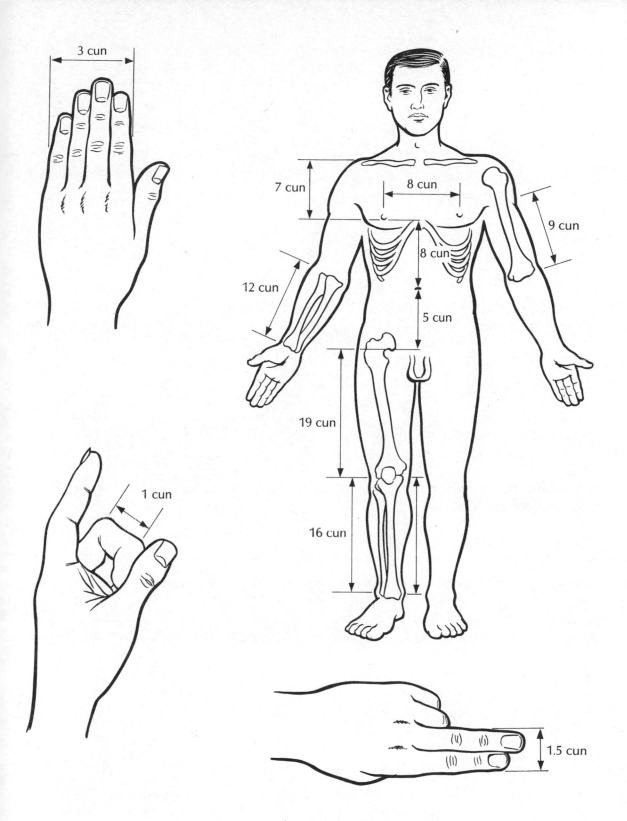

Proportional cun measurements.

6.

Ear Acupuncture

The ear has all the organs and tissues of the body represented on it. In China, ear acupuncture is occasionally used to treat internal disease, but is much more frequently used for the treatment of pain and as a method of providing analgesia. The current Chinese methods of ear acupuncture are not well suited to the treatment of internal disease. The best approach for treating such problems has been defined by Dr Paul Nogier of Lyon, France. The most comprehensive English text discussing auricular therapy and auricular medicine is that written by Dr Julian Kenyon (*Modern Techniques of Acupuncture Volume II,* 1983, Thorsons Publishers). Dr Nogier's methods do not fall within the remit of traditional Chinese medicine and therefore rather than embark on the discussion of completely new techniques I have limited myself to a traditional Chinese approach for the treatment of internal disease.

PART TWO: THE DISEASES

7.

Arthritis

ARTHRITIS (Inflammatory Arthropathies)

All types of arthritis are diseases of *bi*; bi means a blocked or obstructed channel. There are several different types of bi within traditional Chinese medicine which encompass the symptom complexes found in many of the inflammatory arthropathies such as *rheumatoid arthritis, Reiter's disease, ankylosing spondylitis, palandromic rheumatism,* etc.

If pain wanders then it is called a *wandering bi,* an inflamed joint causes *hot bi* and a heavy feeling is called *heavy bi*. The common types of arthritis (bi) are: *painful heavy bi, wandering hot bi* and *painful bi. Painful heavy bi* presents with swollen sore joints and chronic malaise. The tongue coating is thin, white and greasy, the tongue proper is pale and tooth-marked and the pulse is forceless. The pathogens invading are *cold* and *damp;* local heat should be used around the affected joints. *Wandering hot bi* is an acute inflammatory arthropathy, such as acute rheumatoid arthritis. The patient complains of fever and painful red swollen joints associated with limited joint movement, morning stiffness and a general lack of mobility. The tongue coating is yellow and greasy and the pulse rapid. *Painful bi* is often a monoarthritis caused by local damage or disruption to the channels. The most common invading pathogen is cold and local heat should be used; the pulse and tongue are frequently normal.

Point Selection

Cold bi
If cold is the invading pathogen local heat *must* be applied to the painful joints. General points of tonification can be used to disperse cold, these include:

LI4. Dispels wind and cold.

Ren6 and St36 are points of general tonification and strengthen the body.

Sp10. Tonifies the blood and disperses cold (the pi-spleen commands the blood).

If the patient is particularly susceptible to invasion by cold then St36 should be treated with moxa.

Hot bi
Du14 and LI11 disperse heat.

Sp6 and Sp9 resolve damp and clear heat (invasion by heat is often associated with invasion by phlegm and damp).

SJ6. Removes any heat present in the sanjiao.

GB39. Is the influential point for the marrow and tonifies the blood.

Painful bi
Use local tender points in or around the joints and distal points on the channels crossing the painful region. The local tender points that occur commonly are:
a) Neck pain, GB20, GB21 and Du14.
b) Shoulder pain, LI15, LI14 and SJ14.
c) Elbow pain, LI11 and H3.
d) Wrist pain, SJ4, SJ5 and LI5.
e) Hip pain, GB29, GB30 and St31.
f) Sciatica, GB30, and treat the distribution of the pain (commonly either down the urinary bladder channel or the gall-bladder channel).
g) Knee pain, Sp9, UB40 and Xiyan (Extra).
h) Ankle pain, St41, GB40 and UB60.

Point Location

LI4.　　In the middle of the first metacarpal on the radial aspect.

LI5.　　On the radial side of the wrist, in the anatomical snuff-box.

LI11.　　Midway between the lateral epicondyle and the lateral aspect of the cubital (elbow) crease, with the elbow flexed.

LI14.　　On the radial side of the humerus, at the insertion of the deltoid.

LI15.　　Antero-inferior to the acromion, in the middle of the upper portion of the deltoid.

St31.　　Directly below the anterior superior iliac spine in the depression on the lateral side of the sartorius, when the thigh is flexed.

St36.　　3 cun below the lateral aspect of the knee joint line, one finger's breadth from the anterior crest of the tibia.

St41.　　At the junction of the dorsum of the foot and the leg between the tendons of extensor digitorum longus and hallucis longus.

36

Arthritis

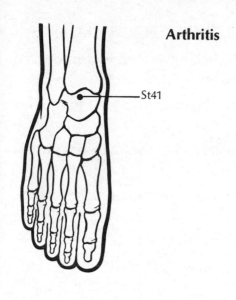

St41

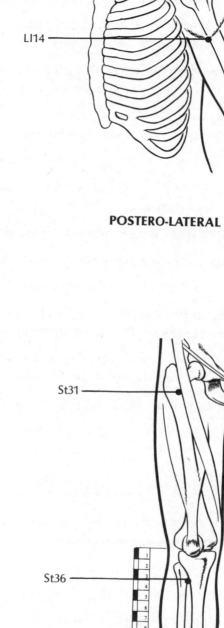

LI15

LI14

POSTERO-LATERAL

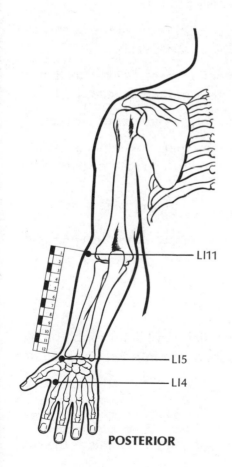

LI11

LI5

LI4

POSTERIOR

St31

St36

ANTERIOR

Sp6.   3 cun above the medial malleolus just posterior to the tibial border.

Sp9.   On the lower border of the medial condyle of the tibia, in the depression between the posterior border of the tibia and the gastrocnemius.

Sp10. 2 cun above the mediosuperior border of the patella on the bulge of the medial portion of the quadriceps femoris.

H3.   When the elbow is flexed this point is at the medial end of the transverse cubital crease, in the depression anterior to the medial epicondyle of the humerus.

UB40. The mid point of the transverse crease of the popliteal fossa between the tendons of biceps femoris and semitendinosus.

UB60. In the depression between the lateral malleolus and the tendo-calcaneus.

SJ4.   At the junction of the ulna and carpal bones, in a depression lateral to the extensor digitorum communis.

SJ5.   2 cun above the posterior wrist crease between the radius and the ulna.

SJ6.   3 cun above the medial wrist crease between the ulna and radius.

SJ14. Posterior and inferior to the acromion, 1 cun posterior to LI15.

GB20. In the posterior aspect of the neck, below the occipital bone, in the depression between the upper portion of sternocleidomastoid and trapezius.

GB21. Midway between the acromion and the vertebral prominence of C7; insert this needle obliquely into the body of the trapezius, do not insert it perpendicularly.

GB29. Midway between the anterior superior iliac spine and the greater trochanter.

GB30. At the junction of the middle and lateral third of a line joining the greater trochanter and the sacral hiatus; puncture with a three-inch needle deep into the pyriformis.

GB39. 3 cun above the tip of the lateral malleolus in the depression between the posterior border of the fibula and the tendons of peroneus longus and brevis.

GB40. Anterior and inferior to the external malleolus in the depression on the lateral side of the tendon of extensor digitorum longus.

Du14. In the mid-line between the transverse process of C7 and T1.

Ren6. 1.5 cun below the umbilicus in the mid-line.

Xiyan (Extra). A pair of points in the two depressions medial and lateral to the patella ligaments, located with the knee flexed; needles should be inserted with the knee flexed.

Treatment Note:
If there is an acute inflammatory arthritis *do not* place needles into the joints as this may

Arthritis

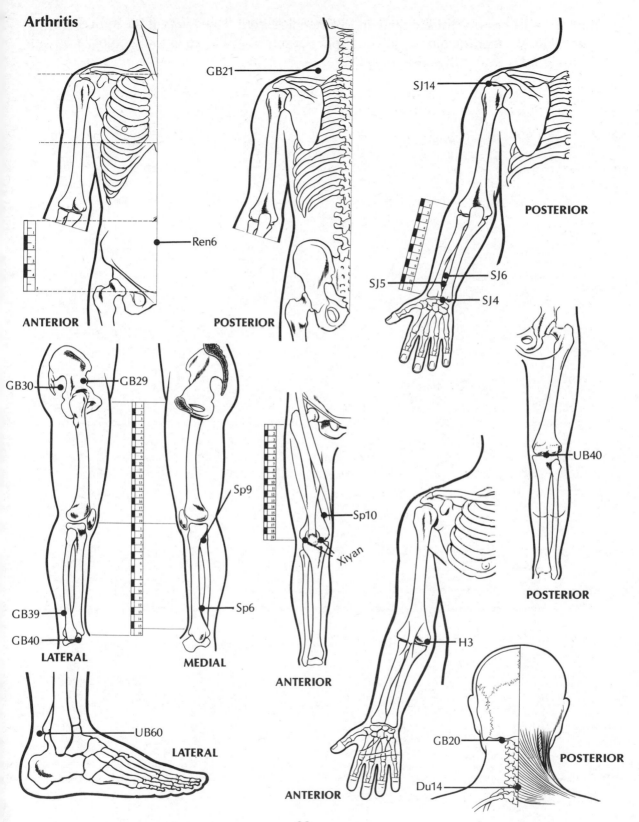

ANTERIOR

GB21

POSTERIOR

Ren6

SJ14

SJ5 SJ6 SJ4

POSTERIOR

GB30 GB29

Sp9

Sp10

Xiyan

UB40

POSTERIOR

GB39
GB40

LATERAL

Sp6

MEDIAL

ANTERIOR

H3

UB60

LATERAL

GB20

Du14

POSTERIOR

ANTERIOR

39

flare the arthropathy; treat local pain with needles around the joints. If the joint is cold but painful insert needles into the joints. If pain or symptoms relating to the joints are worse during cold weather then use local moxa.

8.

Cardiovascular and Chest Diseases

ANGINA PECTORIS

In general terms coronary artery disease is caused by emotional disturbance, inadequate diet (including over-indulgence) and a lack of exercise. Within traditional Chinese medicine there are four main causes of angina:

1. Shi type (retardation of blood and stagnation of qi)
This presents with paroxysmal attacks of angina with a fixed painful area usually over the left shoulder, but pain can occur over the whole back. The patient usually has cold extremities, is pale and cyanosed. The tongue proper is purple and the tongue coating is thin and white with a bowstring or irregular pulse.

2. Shi type (obstruction by phlegm and stagnant blood)
This presents with a stuffy suffocating feeling in the chest and paroxysmal attacks of angina. The tongue proper is purple, the tongue coating is white and greasy and the pulse is bowstring.

3. Xu type (xu of yin of gan-liver and shen-kidney)
This presents with dizziness, thirst, a stuffy feeling in the chest and lumbar discomfort. The tongue coating is thin, the pulse bowstring and thready.

4. Xu type (xu of yang of xin-heart and shen-kidney)
This presents with palpitations, dyspnoea, attacks of angina, malaise, pallor, peripheral cyanosis and lumbar discomfort. The tongue proper is light or dark purple and the pulse is thready.

41

Therapy in the shi types should be directed at invigorating the circulation of qi and blood and resolving the obstruction to the channels. In the xu types tonify the deficiency, invigorate the circulation of blood and qi and remove obstruction to the channels.

Point Selection

1. Shi types

Ren17. Invigorates the circulation of qi and blood.

P4. This can be used for symptomatic treatment of acute angina.

P6. Resolves stasis and removes the obstruction to blood flow.

UB14. Back shu point for the pericardium (circulation).

UB17. Back shu point for invigorating the circulation of blood and qi.

St40. For dispersing damp and phlegm.

2. Xu types

a) Xu of gan-liver and shen-kidney.

UB18. Back shu point; tonifies the gan-liver.

UB23. Back shu point; tonifies the shen-kidney.

P6. Resolves stasis and removes the obstruction to blood flow.

Sp6. Tonifies the gan-liver and shen-kidney.

Ren17. Invigorates the circulation of qi and blood.

b) Xu of yang of xin-heart and shen-kidney.

UB14. Back shu point for the pericardium (circulation).

UB23. Back shu point; tonifies the shen-kidney.

P6. Resolves stasis and removes the obstruction to blood flow.

Ren6. Point of general tonification (the Chinese name for this point is sea of qi).

K3. Invigorates the shen-kidney.

Point Location

St40. 8 cun superior and anterior to the lateral malleolus, two fingers' breadth lateral to the tibial crest.

Sp6. 3 cun above the medial malleolus just posterior to the tibial border.

UB14. 1.5 cun lateral to the lower border of the spinous process of T4.

UB17. 1.5 cun lateral to the lower border of the spinous process of T7.

Angina Pectoris

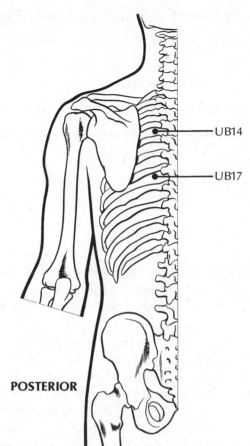

UB14

UB17

POSTERIOR

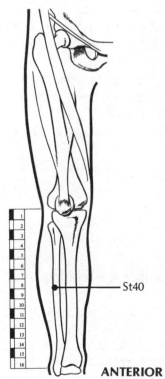

St40

ANTERIOR

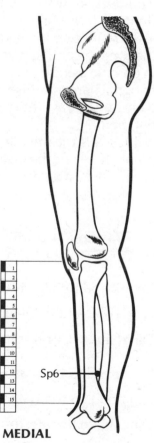

Sp6

MEDIAL

43

UB18. 1.5 cun lateral to the lower border of the spinous process of T9.

UB23. 1.5 cun lateral to the lower border of the spinous process of L2.

K3.   Midway between the top of the medial malleolus and the tendo-calcaneus, level with the tip of the medial malleolus.

P4.   5 cun above the transverse wrist crease (medial) between the radius and ulna.

P6.   2 cun above the transverse wrist crease (medial) between the radius and ulna.

Ren6. 1.5 cun below the umbilicus in the mid-line.

Ren17. At the level of the fourth intercostal space in the mid-line on the sternum; insert obliquely.

ASTHMA

Asthma is related to the *fei-lung, pi-spleen* and *shen-kidney*. Invasion by the pathogens *wind* and *heat* or *wind* and *cold* cause stagnation of the qi of the *fei-lung* and this then turns into phlegm. If the *shen-kidney* is deficient (xu) then the intake of clean qi is impaired and phlegm is produced.

If the pathogen *cold* invades, then the patient presents with a tight wheezy chest and a cough with white frothy sputum. The tongue coating is white and the pulse is rapid and floating. If *heat* invades then the symptoms of an acute chest infection superimposed on asthma appear. The sputum will be thick and yellow and there may be an associated fever; the tongue coating is yellow, the tongue proper is red and the pulse is rapid and excessive. In chronic asthma (xu nature) the patient is breathless on minimal exertion and has a feeble cough. There may also be palpitations and/or central cyanosis. The tongue coating is thin, white and greasy, the tongue proper is light and tooth-marked and the pulse is feeble and deficient.

If *cold* is the invading pathogen, the patient requires heat (cupping over the back shu point). If heat is the invading pathogen, the *phlegm* must be resolved and the temperature controlled. In xu asthma the *fei-lung* and *shen-kidney* should be tonified.

Point Selection

1.   Invasion of cold

UB12 and UB13 remove the obstruction and tonify the fei-lung.

Ren17 and Ren22 promote bronchodilation and relax the chest.

Lu9. Tonifies the fei-lung.

Dingchuan (Extra) stops cough, causes bronchodilation and tonifies the fei-lung.

2.   Invasion by heat

Lu5 and Lu6 tonify the fei-lung and clear heat.

Dingchuan (Extra) stops cough, causes bronchodilation and tonifies the fei-lung.

Angina Pectoris

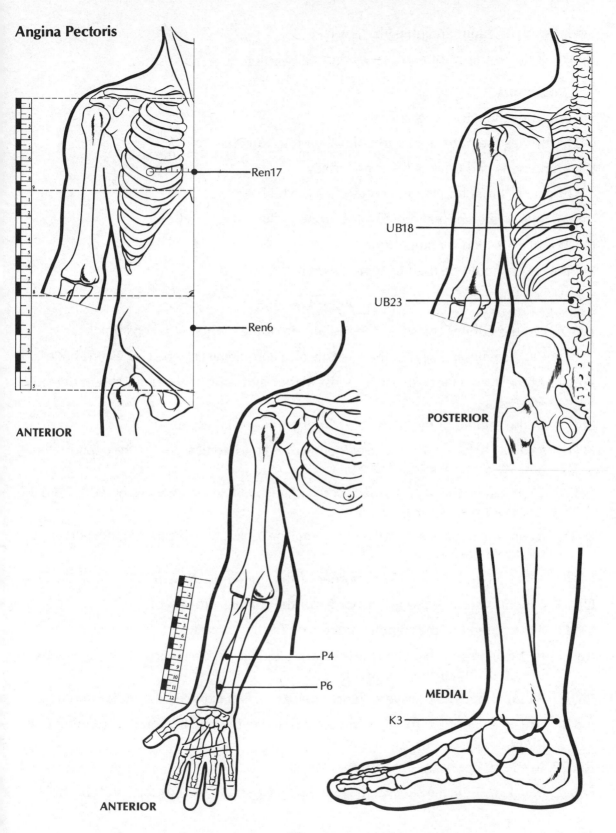

Ren17

Ren6

ANTERIOR

UB18

UB23

POSTERIOR

P4

P6

MEDIAL

K3

ANTERIOR

45

St40. Resolves damp and phlegm.

Ren22. Relaxes the chest and causes bronchodilation.

3.   **Xu asthma**

St36 tonifies the patient generally.

UB43 tonifies the patient, in particular their respiratory system.

K3 strengthens and tonifies the shen-kidney.

UB13 causes bronchodilation and tonifies the fei-lung.

Ren17 relaxes the chest and promotes bronchodilation.

P6 should be added for palpitations.

LI4 and LI11 should be used to bring down fever.

Point Location

Lu5.   On the cubital crease, at the radial side of the tendon at biceps brachii.

Lu6.   On the palmar aspect of the forearm, on a line joining Lu9 and Lu5, 7 cun above Lu9.

Lu9.   At the transverse crease of the wrist, in the depression on the radial side of the radial artery.

LI4.   In the middle of the first metacarpal on the radial aspect.

LI11.   Midway between the lateral epicondyle and the lateral aspect of the cubital (elbow) crease, with the elbow flexed.

St36.   3 cun below the lateral aspect of the knee joint line, one finger's breadth from the anterior crest of the tibia.

St40.   8 cun superior and anterior to the lateral malleolus, two fingers' breadth lateral from the tibial crest.

UB12.   1.5 cun lateral to the lower border of the spinous process of T2.

UB13.   1.5 cun lateral to the lower border of the spinous process of T3.

UB43.   3 cun lateral to the spinous process of T4.

K3.   In the depression between the medial malleolus and the tendo-calcaneus, level with the tip of the medial malleolus.

P6.   2 cun above the transverse wrist crease (medial) between the radius and ulna.

Ren17. At the level of the fourth intercostal space in the mid-line on the sternum; insert obliquely.

Ren22. In the centre of the suprasternal fossa.

Dingchuan (Extra). On the back, at the junction of C7 and T1, 0.5 cun lateral to the mid-line.

Asthma

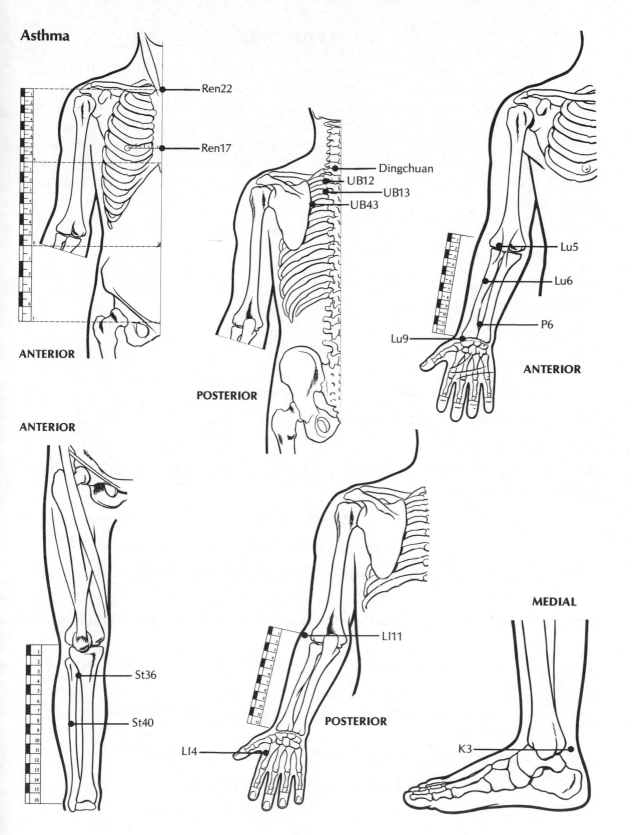

ANTERIOR

Ren22
Ren17

POSTERIOR

Dingchuan
UB12
UB13
UB43

ANTERIOR

Lu5
Lu6
P6
Lu9

ANTERIOR

St36
St40

POSTERIOR

LI11
LI4

MEDIAL

K3

47

ACUTE BRONCHITIS

This may be due to invasion by *wind and cold* or *wind and heat*. Invasion by *wind* and *cold* presents with fever, a cough with watery sputum and general malaise. The tongue coating is thin, white and greasy and the pulse rapid and floating. The *fei-lung* is invaded by *wind* and *cold* impairing the normal ascent of qi. Invasion by *wind* and *heat* results in a high fever with a productive cough and yellow or green sputum. The tongue coating is yellow and thin or yellow and greasy, the pulse is rapid and floating. Invasion by *wind* and *cold* equates well with a viral chest infection and invasion by *wind* and *heat* is more likely to be a bacterial chest infection.

Point Selection

1. Wind and cold

UB12 and UB13 free the flow of qi in the fei-lung and resolve the phlegm.

Lu5 and Lu7 tonify the fei-lung.

St40 resolves the phlegm and damp in the fei-lung.

2. Wind and heat

UB12, UB13 and Lu9 free the flow of qi in the fei-lung.

Du14 and LI11 resolve the pathogen heat.

St40 eliminates damp.

In diseases of cold it is important to warm with moxa or cupping; the back shu points should be treated with cupping.

Point Location

Lu5. On the cubital crease, at the radial side of the tendon at biceps brachii.

Lu7. Superior to the styloid process of the radius, 1.5 cun above the transverse crease of the wrist.

Lu9. At the transverse crease of the wrist, in the depression on the radial side of the radial artery.

LI11. Midway between the lateral epicondyle and the lateral aspect of the cubital (elbow) crease, with the elbow flexed.

St40. 8 cun superior and anterior to the lateral malleolus, two fingers' breadth lateral from the tibial crest.

UB12. 1.5 cun lateral to the lower border of the spinous process of T2.

UB13. 1.5 cun lateral to the lower border of the spinous process of T3.

Du14. In the mid-line between the transverse process of C7 and T1.

Acute Bronchitis

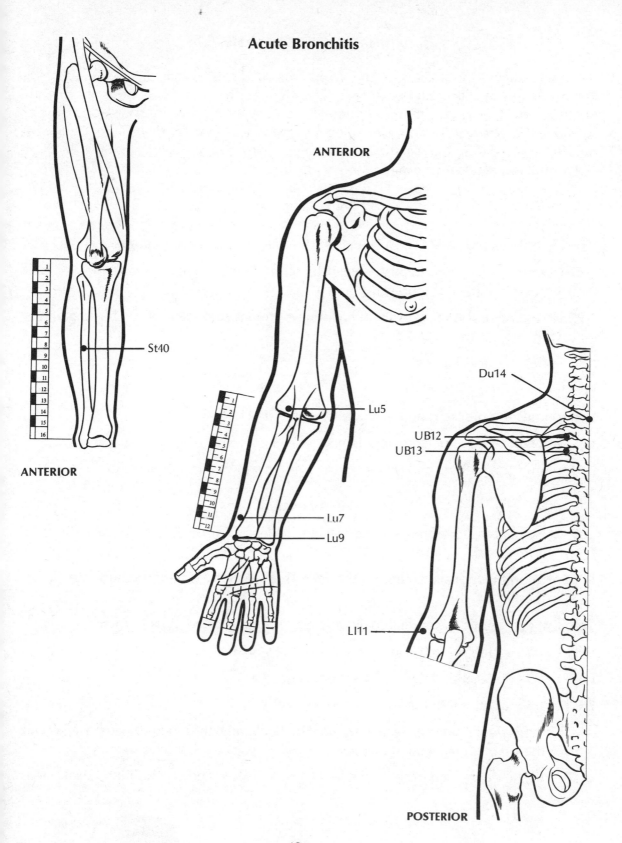

ANTERIOR

ANTERIOR

POSTERIOR

St40

Lu5

Lu7

Lu9

Du14

UB12

UB13

LI11

CHRONIC BRONCHITIS

Acupuncture can only alleviate the symptoms of chronic bronchitis, particularly the accumulation of *phlegm* and any reversible element that there may be in the airways obstruction. Three organs may be affected by chronic bronchitis: the *shen-kidney*, the *pi-spleen* or the *gan-liver*. Therapy should be directed at tonifying the *shen-kidney* and/or the *pi-spleen* or sedating the *gan-liver* depending on which organs seem to have the most functional impairment on examination.

Point Selection

UB13 is the back shu point of the fei-lung, and tonifies this organ, promoting bronchodilation.

UB20 is the back shu point of the pi-spleen. If cold or damp are present then cupping should be used over the back shu point.

UB23 is the back shu point of the shen-kidney; prolonged disease of the fei-lung almost invariably affects the shen-kidney.

K3 tonifies the shen-kidney.

Liv3 sedates the gan-liver.

Sp6 tonifies the pi-spleen and promotes the function of St40.

St40 is the pathogens phlegm and damp.

Lu9 tonifies the fei-lung and promotes the free flow of qi through this organ.

Point Location

Lu9.   At the transverse crease of the wrist, in the depression on the radial side of the radial artery.

St40.   8 cun superior and anterior to the lateral malleolus, two fingers' breadth lateral from the tibial crest.

Sp6.   3 cun above the medial malleolus just posterior to the tibial border.

UB13.   1.5 cun lateral to the lower border of the spinous process of T3.

UB20.   1.5 cun lateral to the spinous process of T11.

UB23.   1.5 cun lateral to the spinous process of L2.

K3.   In the depression between the medial malleolus and the tendo-calcaneus, level with the tip of the medial malleolus.

Liv3.   In the depression distal to the junction of the first and second metatarsal bones.

Chronic Bronchitis

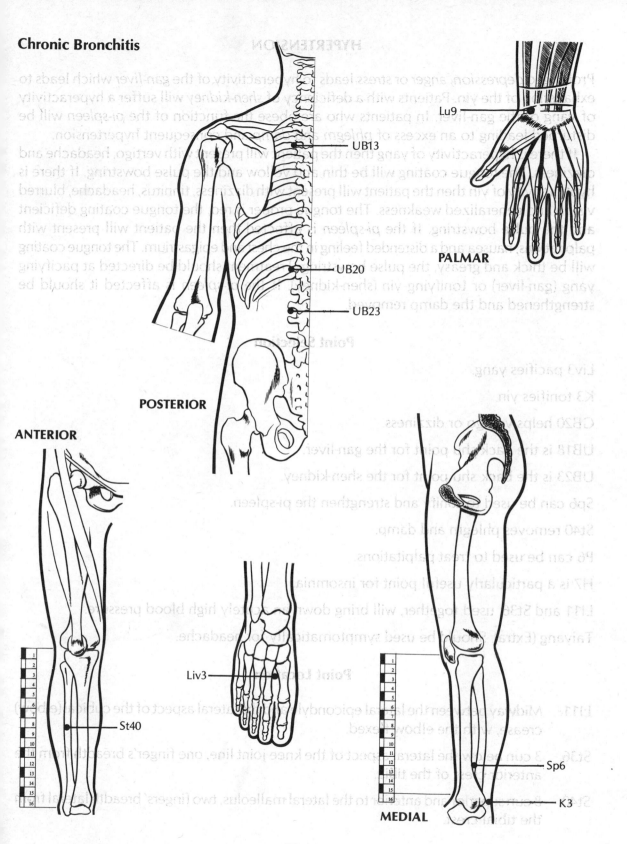

POSTERIOR

UB13

UB20

UB23

PALMAR

Lu9

ANTERIOR

St40

Liv3

MEDIAL

Sp6

K3

HYPERTENSION

Prolonged *depression, anger* or *stress* leads to hyperactivity of the *gan-liver* which leads to exhaustion of the yin. Patients with a deficiency of *shen-kidney* will suffer a hyperactivity of yang of the gan-liver. In patients who are obese the function of the *pi-spleen* will be disturbed leading to an excess of *phlegm* and *damp* and consequent hypertension.

If there is hyperactivity of yang then the patient will present with vertigo, headache and dizziness. The tongue coating will be thin and yellow and the pulse bowstring. If there is hyperactivity of yin then the patient will present with dizziness, tinnitus, headache, blurred vision and generalized weakness. The tongue proper is red, the tongue coating deficient and the pulse bowstring. If the *pi-spleen* is affected then the patient will present with palpitations, nausea and a distended feeling in the chest and epigastrium. The tongue coating will be thick and greasy, the pulse bowstring. Treatment should be directed at pacifying yang (gan-liver) or tonifying yin (shen-kidney). If the *pi-spleen* is affected it should be strengthened and the damp removed.

Point Selection

Liv3 pacifies yang.

K3 tonifies yin.

GB20 helps vertigo or dizziness.

UB18 is the back shu point for the gan-liver.

UB23 is the back shu point for the shen-kidney.

Sp6 can be used to tonify and strengthen the pi-spleen.

St40 removes phlegm and damp.

P6 can be used to treat palpitations.

H7 is a particularly useful point for insomnia.

LI11 and St36, used together, will bring down an acutely high blood pressure.

Taiyang (Extra). Should be used symptomatically for headache.

Point Location

LI11.   Midway between the lateral epicondyle and the lateral aspect of the cubical (elbow) crease, with the elbow flexed.

St36.   3 cun below the lateral aspect of the knee joint line, one finger's breadth from the anterior crest of the tibia.

St40.   8 cun superior and anterior to the lateral malleolus, two fingers' breadth lateral from the tibial crest.

Hypertension

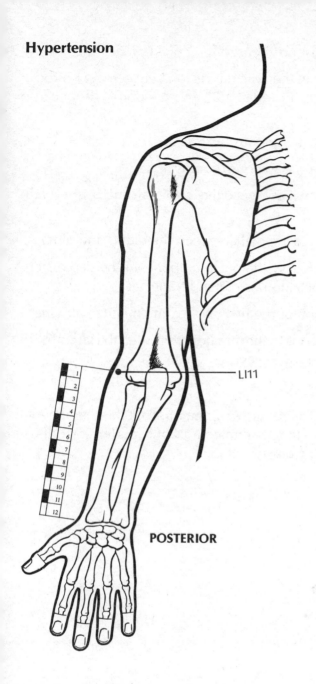

LI11

POSTERIOR

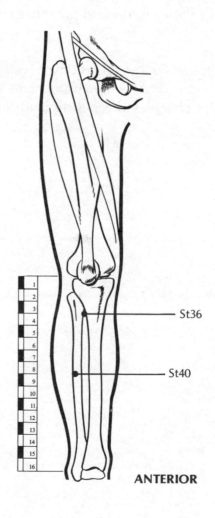

St36

St40

ANTERIOR

53

Sp6. 3 cun above the medial malleolus just posterior to the tibial border.

H7. On the transverse crease of the wrist in the articular region between the pisiform bone and the ulna, in the depression on the radial side of the tendon of flexor carpi ulnaris.

UB18. 1.5 cun lateral to the lower border of the spinous process of T9.

UB23. 1.5 cun lateral to the lower border of the spinous process of L2.

K3. In the depression between the medial malleolus and the tendo-calcaneus, level with the tip of the medial malleolus.

P6. 2 cun above the transverse wrist crease (medial) between the radius and ulna.

GB20. In the posterior aspect of the neck, below the occipital bone, in the depression between the upper portion of sternocleidomastoid and trapezius.

Liv3. In the depression distal to the junction of the first and second metatarsal bones.

Taiyang (Extra). In the depression 1 cun posterior to the mid-point between the lateral end of the eyebrow and the outer canthus of the eye.

Note:

The symptoms of hypertension are well controlled with acupuncture, but this therapeutic modality does not seem to produce effective longer-term control of hypertension unless treatment is repeated very frequently (every week or two).

Hypertension

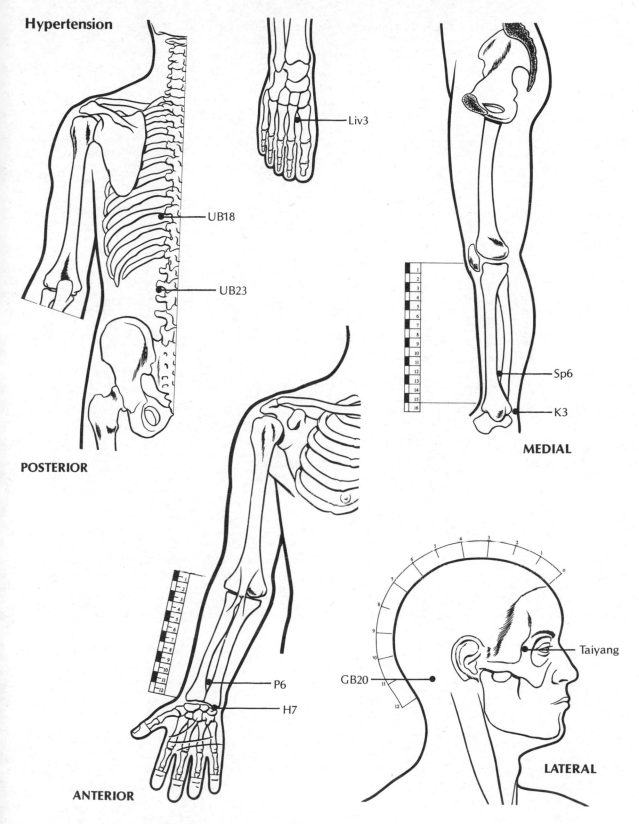

Liv3

UB18

UB23

POSTERIOR

Sp6

K3

MEDIAL

P6

H7

Taiyang

GB20

LATERAL

ANTERIOR

55

9.

Gastrointestinal Diseases

ABDOMINAL PAIN (Irritable Bowel, Spastic Colon)

Undiagnosed abdominal pain (within the paradigms of conventional medicine) is a common problem. It's often called irritable bowel or spastic colon, but this usually represents no more than a convenient diagnostic label for a largely undiagnosed group of patients. In traditional Chinese terms this may be caused by accumulation of *cold* or by the retardation of the qi of the *pi-spleen* impairing the function of the *pi-spleen* and *stomach*. In internal accumulation of *cold* the patient will present with sudden violent crampy abdominal pain which responds to warmth. They will have loose stools, a white coated tongue and a deep forceful pulse. Dysfunction of the *pi-spleen* presents with epigastric and abdominal distension and pain which is aggravated by pressure. The patient often has excessive flatulence and an acid feeling in their mouth; the pain may be accompanied by diarrhoea and relieved after defaecation. The tongue coating is greasy and the pulse deficient.

Point selection

1. **Invasion by cold**
    Sp10 tonifies the blood and disperses cold.

    St36 and Ren6 tonify and strengthen the body.

    Use local heat (cupping or moxa) over the painful area.

2. **Dysfunction of the pi-spleen**
    Sp6 tonifies the pi-spleen.

    St36 acts with Sp6 to strengthen its function and invigorates the qi of the stomach.

St40 disperses the pathogen phlegm and damp; dysfunction of the pi-spleen often leads to invasion of the pathogen damp.

P6 should be used if there is nausea or vomiting present.

St25 is the front mu point for the large intestine and should be used if there is colonic dysfunction.

Local tender points should be used over the abdomen; one inch needles should be inserted into the tender point.

Distal points should be used on the channel crossing the painful area (St44 and Sp6).

Point Location

St25.   2 cun lateral to the navel.

St36.   3 cun below the lateral aspect of the knee joint line, one finger's breadth from the anterior crest of the tibia.

St40.   8 cun superior and anterior to the lateral malleolus, two fingers' breadth lateral from the tibial crest.

St44.   Proximal to the web margin between the second and third toes in the depression distal and lateral to the second metatarso digital joint.

Sp6.   3 cun above the medial malleolus just posterior to the tibial border.

Sp10.   2 cun above the mediosuperior border of the patella on the bulge of the medial portion of the quadriceps femoris.

P6.   2 cun above the transverse crease to the wrist between the tendons of palmaris longus and flexor carpi radialis.

Ren6.   1.5 cun below the umbilicus in the mid-line.

Note:
A diagnosis as to the cause of the abdominal pain should *always* be made prior to treating with acupuncture. Acupuncture should *only* be used after the need for acute medical or surgical management has been considered.

Abdominal Pain

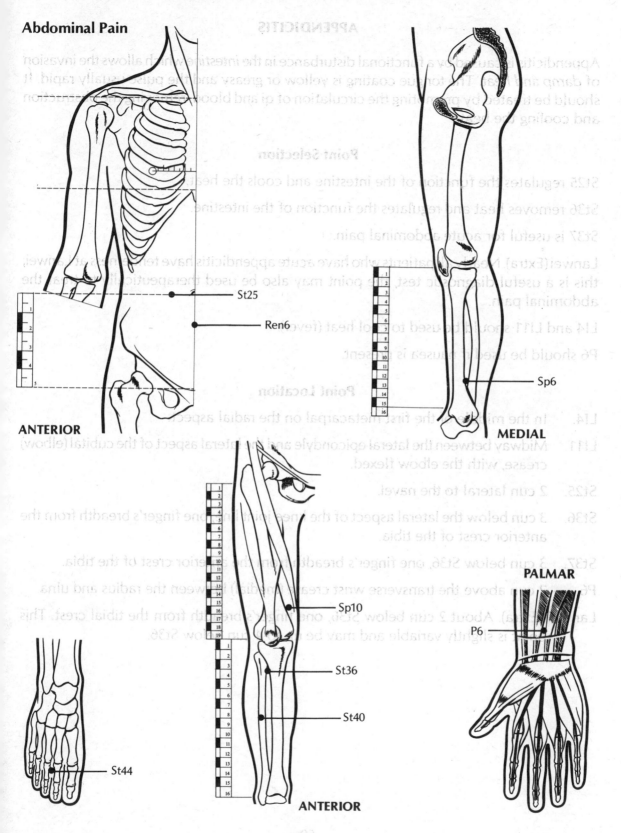

ANTERIOR

St25

Ren6

MEDIAL

Sp6

PALMAR

P6

Sp10

St36

St40

ANTERIOR

St44

59

APPENDICITIS

Appendicitis is caused by a functional disturbance in the *intestine* which allows the invasion of *damp and heat*. The tongue coating is yellow or greasy and the pulse usually rapid. It should be treated by promoting the circulation of qi and blood, removing the obstruction and cooling the heat.

Point Selection

St25 regulates the function of the intestine and cools the heat.

St36 removes heat and regulates the function of the intestine.

St37 is useful for acute abdominal pain.

Lanwei (Extra). Nearly all patients who have acute appendicitis have tenderness at Lanwei; this is a useful diagnostic test, the point may also be used therapeutically to treat the abdominal pain.

LI4 and LI11 should be used to cool heat (fever).

P6 should be used if nausea is present.

Point Location

LI4.   In the middle of the first metacarpal on the radial aspect.

LI11.   Midway between the lateral epicondyle and the lateral aspect of the cubital (elbow) crease, with the elbow flexed.

St25.   2 cun lateral to the navel.

St36.   3 cun below the lateral aspect of the knee joint line, one finger's breadth from the anterior crest of the tibia.

St37.   3 cun below St36, one finger's breadth from the anterior crest of the tibia.

P6.   2 cun above the transverse wrist crease (medial) between the radius and ulna.

Lanwei (Extra). About 2 cun below St36, one finger's breadth from the tibial crest. This point is slightly variable and may be up to 4 cun below St36.

Appendicitis

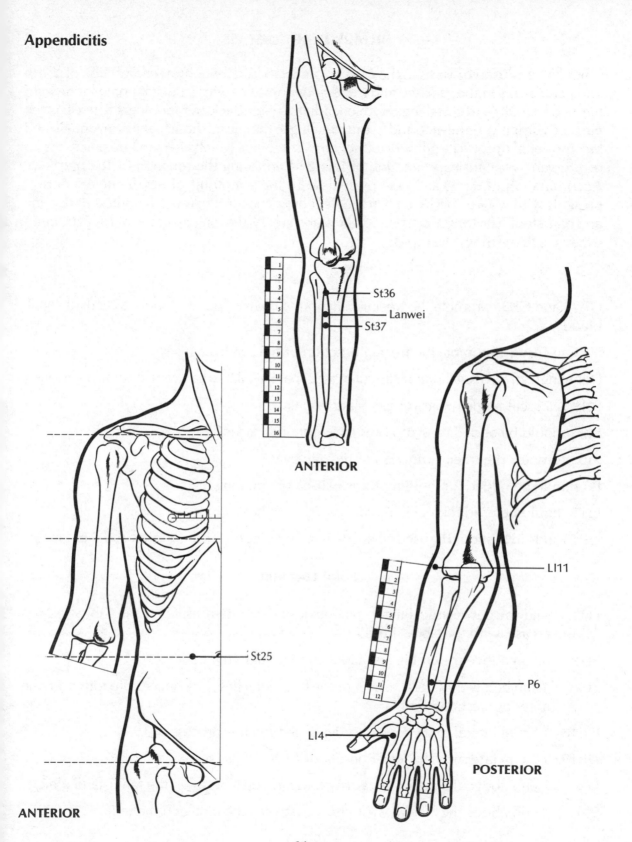

St36

Lanwei

St37

ANTERIOR

LI11

P6

LI4

St25

ANTERIOR

POSTERIOR

61

This can be caused by stasis in the *gan-liver* and *gall-bladder* or by accumulation of *damp* and *heat*. Stasis in the *gan-liver* and *gall-bladder* presents with a bursting pain in the right hypochondrium and costal region which radiates to the back and shoulders. There is often nausea, vomiting, flatulence and a stuffy feeling in the chest. These feelings are intensified by emotional upset. The primary pathogen is irritability, which alters the freeing function of the *gan-liver* causing stagnation of bile and impairing the function of the *pi-spleen*. Accumulation of *damp* and *heat* presents with the symptoms of acute cholecystitis. It presents with severe colicky pain in the right hypochondrium, fever, jaundice, dark urine and pale stool. The tongue coating is yellow and greasy, the tongue proper red and the pulse excessive (bowstring) and rapid.

Point Selection

GB24 and GB34 promote the freeing function of the gan-liver and more directly the gall-bladder.

Liv3 and Liv 14 promote the freeing function of the gan-liver.

Dannang(Extra) is usually tender in gall-bladder pain, similar to Lanwei(Extra) in appendicitis.

St19 is a local tender point for gall-bladder pain.

St36 should be added for symptoms of abdominal distension.

SJ6 promotes the freeing function of the gan-liver.

P6 should be added for the symptoms nausea or vomiting.

LI11 should be used for fever, in order to disperse heat.

UB18 and UB19 should be used where there is jaundice or pain referred to the shoulder tip.

Point Location

LI11.   Midway between the lateral epicondyle and the lateral aspect of the cubital (elbow) crease, with the elbow flexed.

St19.   6 cun above the umbilicus, and 2 cun lateral to the mid-line.

St36.   3 cun below the lateral aspect of the knee joint line, one finger's breadth from the anterior crest of the tibia.

UB18. 1.5 cun lateral to the lower border of the spinous process of T9.

UB19. 1.5 cun lateral to the lower border of the spinous process of T10.

P6.   2 cun above the transverse wrist crease (medial) between the radius and ulna.

SJ6.   3 cun above the medial wrist crease between the ulna and the radius.

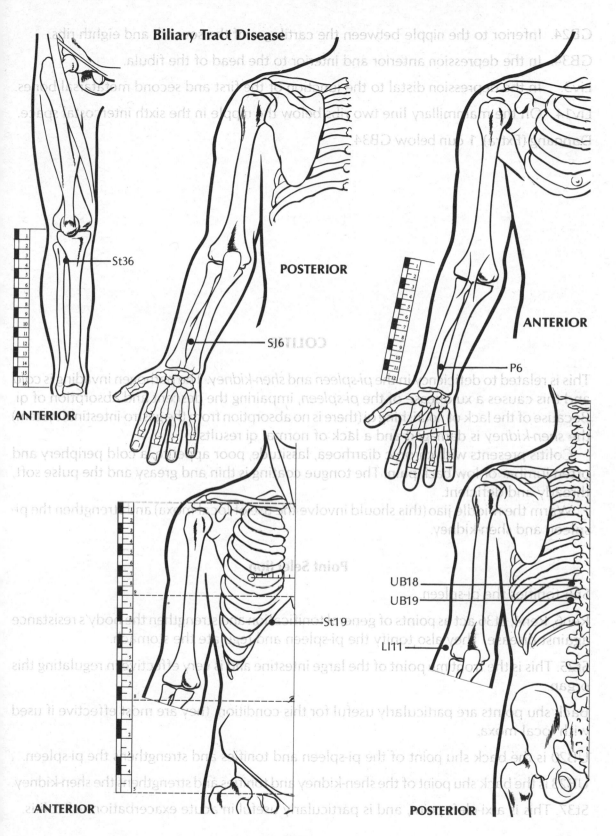

St36

POSTERIOR

SJ6

ANTERIOR

ANTERIOR

P6

St19

UB18

UB19

LI11

ANTERIOR

POSTERIOR

GB24. Inferior to the nipple between the cartilages of the seventh and eighth ribs.

GB34. In the depression anterior and interior to the head of the fibula.

Liv3. In the depression distal to the junction of the first and second metatarsal bones.

Liv14. On the mammillary line two ribs below the nipple in the sixth intercostal space.

Dannang (Extra). 1 cun below GB34.

COLITIS

This is related to deficiency in the *pi-spleen* and *shen-kidney*. The pathogen invading is *cold* and this causes a xu disease of the *pi-spleen*, impairing the descent and absorption of qi. Because of the lack of nourishing qi (there is no absorption from the gastro-intestinal system) the *shen-kidney* is damaged and a lack of normal qi results.

Colitis presents with chronic diarrhoea, lassitude, poor appetite, a cold periphery and often lumbar or low back pain. The tongue coating is thin and greasy and the pulse soft, thready and deficient.

Warm the middle jiao (this should involve the use of local moxa) and strengthen the pi-spleen and shen-kidney.

Point Selection

Sp6 tonifies the pi-spleen.

Ren6, Ren4, St36 act as points of general tonification and strengthen the body's resistance against disease. They also tonify the pi-spleen and regulate the stomach.

St25. This is the front mu point of the large intestine and is very effective in regulating this organ.

Back shu points are particularly useful for this condition, they are most effective if used with local moxa.

UB20 is the back shu point of the pi-spleen and tonifies and strengthens the pi-spleen.

UB23 is the back shu point of the shen-kidney and tonifies and strengthens the shen-kidney.

St37. This is a xi-cleft point, and is particularly useful in acute exacerbations of colitis.

Biliary Tract Disease

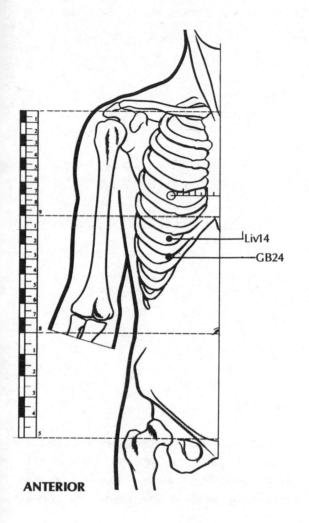

ANTERIOR

Liv14
GB24

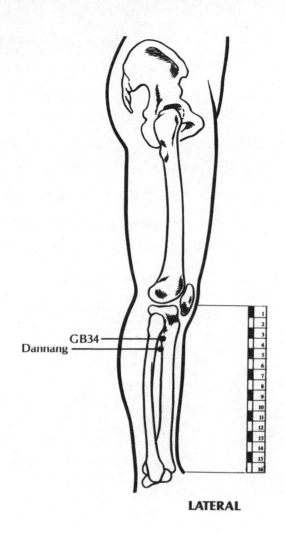

GB34
Dannang

LATERAL

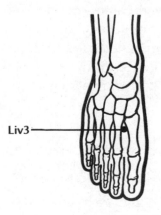

Liv3

65

Point Location

St25. 2 cun lateral to the navel.

St36. 3 cun below the lateral aspect of the knee joint line, one finger's breadth from the anterior crest of the tibia.

St37. 3 cun below St36, one finger's breadth from the anterior crest of the tibia.

Sp6. 3 cun above the medial malleolus just posterior to the tibial border.

UB20. 1.5 cun lateral to the spinous process of T11.

UB23. 1.5 cun lateral to the spinous process of L2.

Ren4. On the mid line of the abdomen 3 cun below the umbilicus.

Ren6. 1.5 cun below the umbilicus in the mid-line.

GASTROENTERITIS

This presents with vomiting, diarrhoea, colicky abdominal pain, fever and headache. The *stomach* and *pi-spleen* are invaded by summer *heat and damp,* or they may be injured by the intake of contaminated food. This damage the digestive functions of the *pi-spleen;* adverse ascent of qi causes vomiting and descent of qi causes diarrhoea. The tongue coating is white and thin or yellow, the pulse rapid and often deficient.

Eliminate *damp* and *heat* and tonify the *pi-spleen* and *stomach.* Acute gastroenteritis should be treated every four hours for thirty minutes at each treatment; treatment should continue until the symptoms clear.

Point Selection

P6 stops adverse ascent of qi (vomiting).

St25, St36 and Ren12 free and regulate the function of the intestine and stomach.

St44 and UB40 eliminate heat and control the body temperature.

Colitis

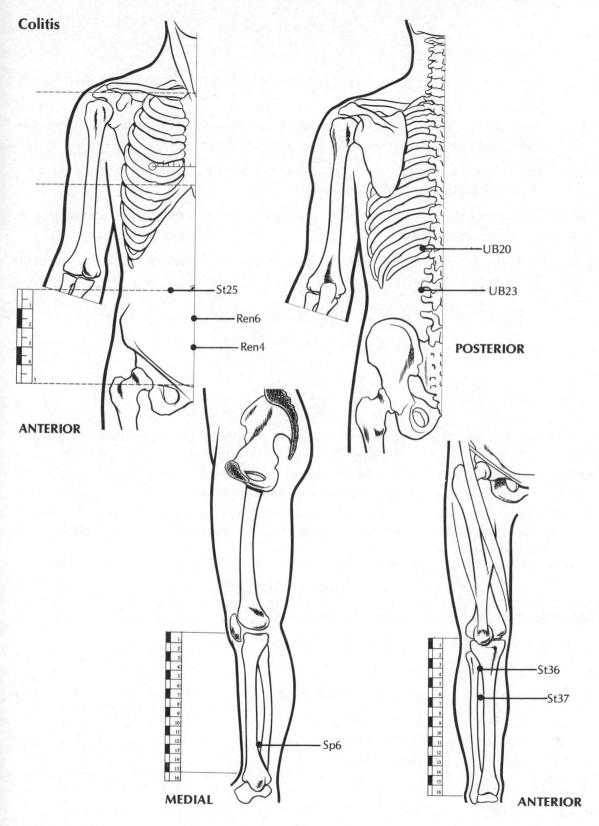

ANTERIOR

St25
Ren6
Ren4

POSTERIOR

UB20
UB23

MEDIAL

Sp6

ANTERIOR

St36
St37

67

St25. 2 cun lateral to the navel.

St36. 3 cun below the lateral aspect of the knee joint line, one finger's breadth from the anterior crest of the tibia.

St44. Proximal to the web margin between the second and third toes in the depression distal and lateral to the second metatarsodigital joint.

UB40. The mid point of the transverse crease of the popliteal fossa between the tendons of biceps femoris and semitendinosus.

P6. 2 cun above the transverse crease to the wrist between the tendons of palmaris longus and flexor carpi radialis.

Ren12. On the mid-line of the abdomen between the naval and the xiphisternum, 4 cun above the umbilicus.

HICCUPS

In traditional Chinese terms hiccups are caused by either failure of the qi of the *stomach* to descend and stagnation of the qi of the *gan-liver*, or adverse ascent of qi of the *stomach* caused by the pathogenic factor *cold*. Stagnation of qi of the *gan-liver* presents with epigastric and abdominal distension, hiccups, a distended feeling in the chest and hypochondrium and irritability. The tongue coating will be yellow and greasy, the pulse forceful. Invasion by the pathogen *cold* presents with slow forceful hiccups alleviated by hot drinks. The tongue coating will be white and the pulse slow.

Point Selection

St36 regulates the function of the stomach.

Ren12 is the influential point for the fu organs and activates qi.

P6 stops the adverse ascent of qi.

UB17 invigorates the circulation of blood and qi.

1. Stagnation of the qi of the gan-liver:
    St44 readjusts the stomach and relieves stagnation.
    Liv3 tonifies the qi of the gan-liver.

2. Invasion by cold:
    Ren13 warms the pi-spleen and stomach and eliminates cold.

Gastroenteritis

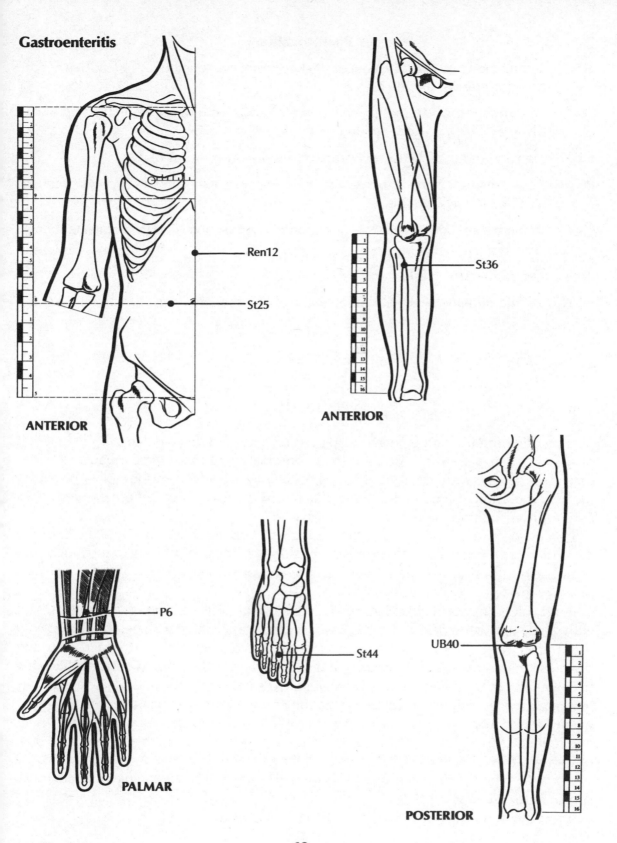

Ren12

St25

ANTERIOR

St36

ANTERIOR

P6

PALMAR

St44

UB40

POSTERIOR

69

Point Location

St36. 3 cun below the lateral aspect of the knee joint line, one finger's breadth from the anterior crest of the tibia.

St44. Proximal to the web margin between the second and third toes in the depression distal and lateral to the second metatarso digital joint.

UB17. 1.5 cun lateral to the lower border of the spinous process of T7.

P6. 2 cun above the transverse crease to the wrist between the tendons of palmaris longus and flexor carpi radialis.

Liv3. In the depression distal to the junction of the first and second metatarsal bones.

Ren12. On the mid-line of the abdomen between the naval and the xiphisternum, 4 cun above the umbilicus.

Ren13. On the mid-line of the abdomen 5 cun above the umbilicus.

PEPTIC ULCER

This usually presents with pain in the epigastric region and may be due to a dysfunction of the *pi-spleen, gan-liver* or *stomach* (or a combination of these three organs). In obese patients or patients with a weak constitution, the pathogen *cold* can invade easily. This causes the accumulation of food in the stomach and affects the functions of the *pi-spleen*. This can result in haematemesis or a perforated ulcer.

Depression or anger may impair the freeing function of the *gan-liver* and the qi of the *gan-liver* can move transversely to invade the *stomach*. Irregular feeding or too much cold or uncooked food upsets the *stomach* and predisposes to invasion of the stomach and *pi-spleen* by a variety of pathogens.

Peptic ulcers can be divided into xu (deficiency) and shi (excess) types. Xu types present with vague epigastric pain which is relieved by food, associated with heartburn and cold extremities. The pain is often relieved by pressure. The tongue coating is thin and white and the pulse thready, weak and forceless. It is usually the *pi-spleen* that is deficient allowing the invasion of the pathogen *cold* which causes a disturbance of the middle jiao and results in a peptic ulcer. Shi ulcers present with a full or bursting epigastric pain, which is worse when pressed and may be associated with irritability, flatulence, restlessness, heartburn and reduced food intake. The tongue coating is thin and white and the pulse excessive or bowstring. This is caused by dysfunction of the *gan-liver*.

In the xu type the *pi-spleen* should be strengthened and the *stomach* regulated; moxa should be used to disperse the cold. In the shi type the freeing function of the *gan-liver* should be promoted and the function of the *stomach* regulated.

Hiccups

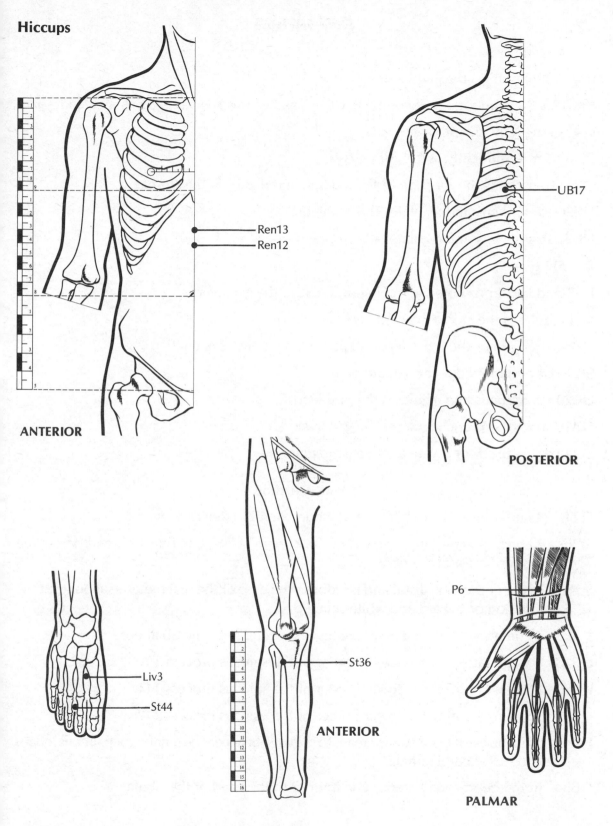

ANTERIOR

Ren13
Ren12

POSTERIOR

UB17

Liv3
St44

ANTERIOR

St36

PALMAR

P6

71

Point Selection

1. Xu type

Ren11 strengthens the pi-spleen.

Ren12 is the influential point of the fu organs and warms and strengthens the middle jiao.

Sp6 strengthens the pi-spleen.

P6 is symptomatically useful for nausea.

St36 strengthens the function of P6 and Sp6 and regulates the stomach.

UB20 strengthens and regulates the pi-spleen.

UB21 strengthens and regulates the stomach.

2. Shi type

Liv3 and Liv14 promote the freeing function of the gan-liver.

Sp4 regulates the stomach and spleen.

GB34 strengthens the function of all points on the liver channel.

St21 has a marked effect on acute pain.

UB20 strengthens and regulates the pi-spleen.

UB18 strengthens and regulates the gan-liver.

St34 can be used for severe acute gastric pain.

Point Location

St21.   4 cun above the umbilicus and 2 cun lateral to Ren12.

St36.   3 cun below the lateral aspect of the knee joint line, one finger's breadth from the anterior crest of the tibia.

Sp4.   In the depression distal and inferior to the base of the first metatarsal bone, at the junction of the red and white skin.

Sp6.   3 cun above the medial malleolus just posterior to the tibial border.

UB18.   1.5 cun lateral to the lower border of the spinous process T9.

UB20.   1.5 cun lateral to the lower border of the spinous process T11.

UB21.   1.5 cun lateral to the lower border of the spinous process T12.

P6.   2 cun above the transverse crease to the wrist between the tendons of palmaris longus and flexor carpi radialis.

GB34.   In the depression anterior and inferior to the head of the fibula.

Peptic Ulcer

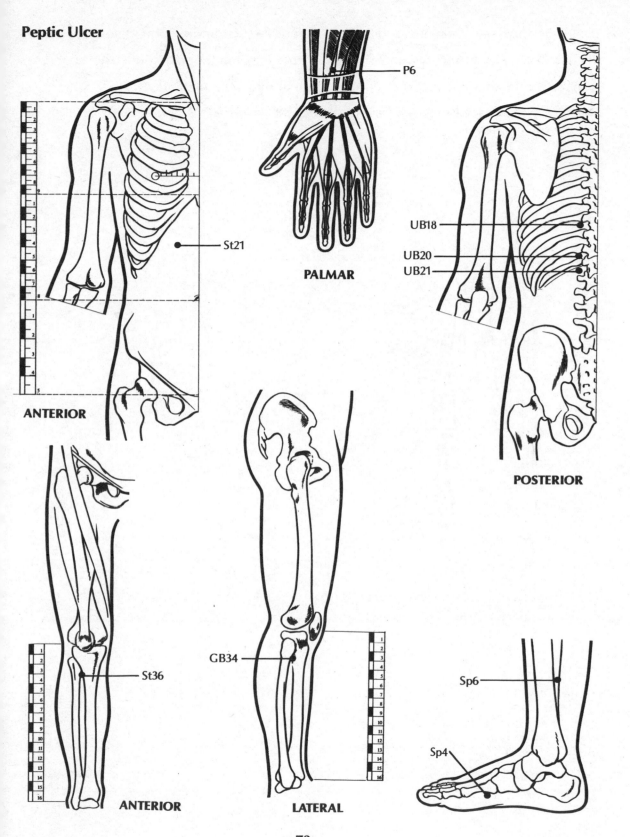

ANTERIOR

PALMAR

P6

St21

POSTERIOR

UB18
UB20
UB21

ANTERIOR

St36

LATERAL

GB34

Sp6

Sp4

Liv3. In the depression distal to the junction of the first and second metatarsal bones.

Liv14. On the mammillary line 2 ribs below the nipple in the sixth intercostal space.

Ren11. On the mid-line of the abdomen 3 cun above the umbilicus.

Ren12. On the mid-line of the abdomen between the navel and the xiphisternum, 4 cun above the umbilicus.

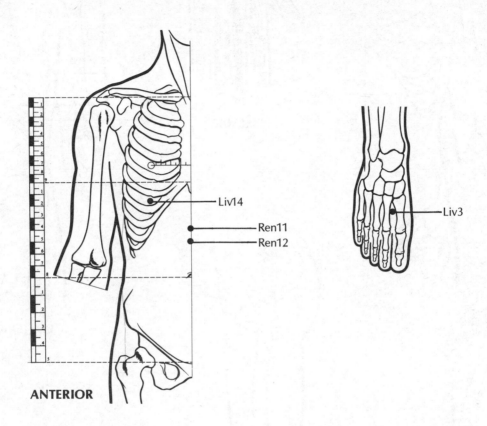

ANTERIOR

10.

Gynaecological and Genito-Urinary Problems

AMENORRHOEA

The main causes of either *stasis* or *exhaustion* of *blood*. Amenorrhoea due to *blood stasis* is caused by mental depression or invasion by the pathogen *cold* during menstruation. Amenorrhoea due to exhaustion of blood results from a deficiency of qi in the liver, spleen and kidney channels which may be caused by a long illness or starvation. Blood stasis usually presents with amenorrhoea of sudden onset and distension and pain in the lower abdomen aggravated by pressure. The tongue is usually normal, the pulse deep and wiry. Blood exhaustion really represents with deficiency of qi in the channels, it presents with delayed menstruation with a menstrual flow that gradually decreases over a number of months leading to amenorrhoea. The patient usually has a sallow complexion, dry skin, anorexia and is listless. The tongue coating is white, the tongue proper pale and tooth-marked and the pulse forceless and deficient.

Point Selection

1.　Blood stasis

Ren3 is the point where the Ren channel and the three yin channels of the foot meet, needling this point promotes the circulation of qi.

Sp6 adjusts the flow of qi and blood.

Sp10 activates blood circulation and promotes menstrual flow.

Liv3 releases the qi of the gan-liver.

St29 and UB32 are local points used to remove blood stasis in the uterus.

LI4 adjusts the flow of qi and blood.

2. Blood exhaustion

Points should be selected to tonify the shen-kidney, pi-spleen and gan-liver.

Ren4 is the point of general tonification.

UB18 is the back shu point of the gan-liver.

UB20 is the back shu point of the pi-spleen.

UB23 is the back shu point of the shen-kidney.

Moxa may be used on all these back shu points.

St25 regulates the pi-spleen and stomach, the sources of qi and blood formation.

St36 is the point of general tonification.

Sp6 is the point where all three yin channels run and can be used to adjust and tonify the flow of qi through the yin channels of the leg.

Point Location

LI4.   In the middle of the first metacarpal on the radial aspect.

St25.   2 cun lateral to the navel.

St29.   4 cun below the umbilicus, 2 cun lateral to the mid-line.

St36.   3 cun below the lateral aspect of the knee joint line, one finger's breadth from the anterior crest of the tibia.

Sp6.   3 cun above the medial malleolus just posterior to the tibial border.

Sp10.   2 cun above the mediosuperior border of the patella on the bulge of the medial portion of the quadriceps femoris.

UB18.   1.5 cun lateral to the lower border of the spinous process of T9.

UB20.   1.5 cun lateral to the spinous process of T11.

UB23.   1.5 cun lateral to the spinous process of L2.

UB32.   In the second posterior sacral foramen, midway between the lower border of the posterior superior iliac spine on the mid-line.

Liv3.   In the depression distal to the junction of the first and second metatarsal bones.

Ren3.   4 cun below the umbilicus and 1 cun above the border of the symphysis pubis, on the mid-line.

Ren4.   On the mid-line of the abdomen 3 cun below the umbilicus.

Amenorrhoea

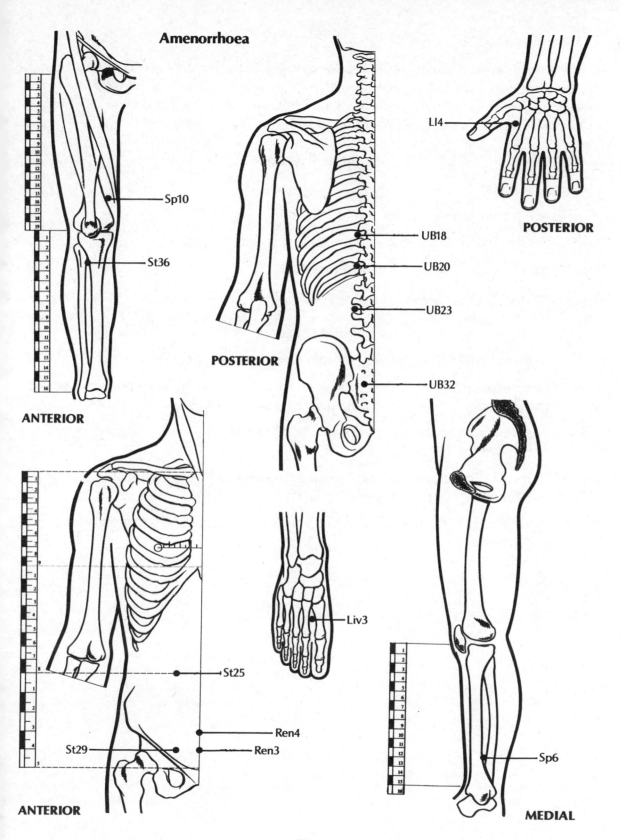

Sp10

St36

ANTERIOR

UB18

UB20

UB23

UB32

POSTERIOR

LI4

POSTERIOR

St25

Ren4

St29

Ren3

ANTERIOR

Liv3

Sp6

MEDIAL

77

CYSTITIS

This is caused by accumulation of *damp and heat* in the *urinary bladder* which disturbs its urinary excretory function. It presents with a frequency of micturition and a burning pain on passing urine. There may be distension in the lower abdomen and in some instances urinary retention. The tongue proper is red with a yellow coating and the pulse is rapid.

Point Selection

LI4 disperses heat.

Ren3 is the front mu point of the urinary bladder channel.

Sp10 activates the channels and collaterals in the bladder region.

UB39 promotes circulation of the water passages.

Sp9 eliminates damp and heat in the urinary bladder.

Point Location

LI4.   In the middle of the first metacarpal on the radial aspect.

Sp9.   On the lower border of the medial condyle of the tibia, in the depression between the posterior border of the tibia and the gastrocnemius.

Sp10.   2 cun above the mediosuperior border of the patella on the bulge of the medial portion of the quadriceps femoris.

UB39.   In the popliteal crease, 1 cun lateral to the middle of the popliteal crease on the medial border of the biceps femoris.

Ren3.   4 cun below the umbilicus and 1 cun above the border of the symphysis pubis, in the mid-line.

Cystitis

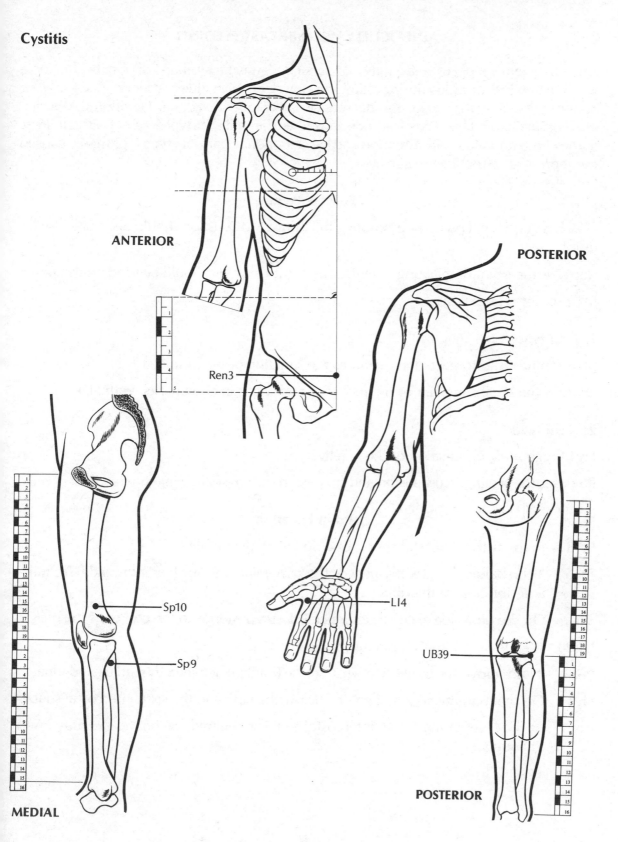

ANTERIOR

POSTERIOR

Ren3

Sp10

Sp9

LI4

UB39

MEDIAL

POSTERIOR

79

DIFFICULTY WITH BREAST FEEDING

An insufficient supply of breast milk can occur because the mother is of poor health, there is a massive loss of blood during childbirth or a depressive illness affecting the *gan-liver*. Xu type presents with a progressive decrease in milk production during lactation, the mother also complains of palpitations, lassitude and rather 'thin' milk. Shi types present with a fullness in the chest, anorexia, milk retention and hypochondriac pain. Shi type is primarily caused by depression affecting the gan-liver.

Point Selection

St18 is a good local point for promoting milk flow. Moxibustion should be applied to this point.

Ren17 is the point dominating qi in the chest. Moxibustion should be used on this point.

SI1 promotes lactation.

1. Xu type

St36 tonifies the stomach and regulates the function of the pi-spleen.

UB20 is the back shu point of the pi-spleen and works in conjunction with St36.

2. Shi type

Liv14 regulates the function of the gan-liver.

P6 eases the feeling of distension and fullness in the chest allowing the free flow of milk.

Point Location

St18.   In the fifth intercostal space, one rib below the nipple.

St36.   3 cun below the lateral aspect of the knee joint line, one finger's breadth from the anterior crest of the tibia.

SI1.   On the ulna side of the little finger, 0.1 cun posterior to the corner of the nail.

UB20. 1.5 cun lateral to the spinous process of T11.

P6.   2 cun above the transverse wrist crease (medial) between the radius and ulna.

Liv14. On the mammillary line two ribs below the nipple in the sixth intercostal space.

Ren17. At the level of the fourth intercostal space in the mid-line on the sternum; insert obliquely.

Difficulty with Breast Feeding

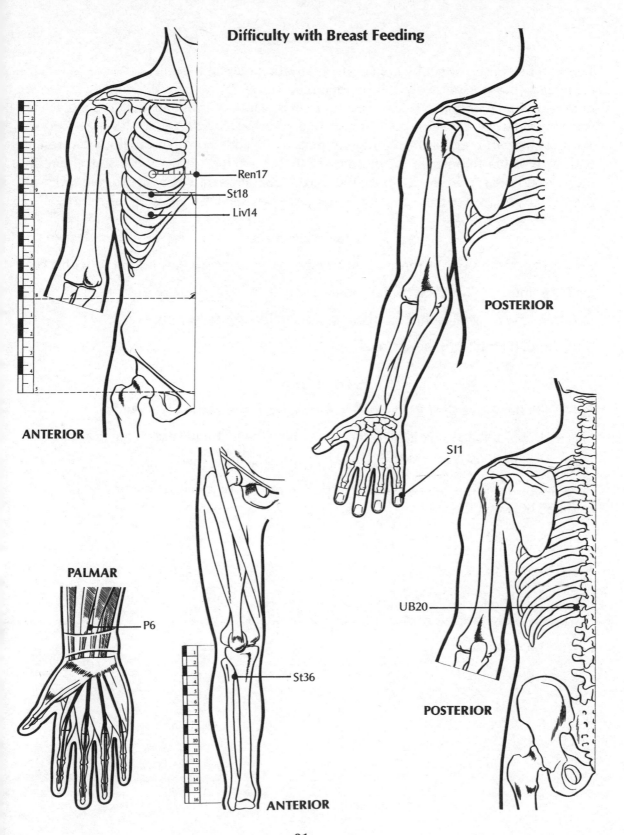

ANTERIOR

Ren17
St18
Liv14

POSTERIOR

SI1

PALMAR

P6

St36

ANTERIOR

UB20

POSTERIOR

81

DYSMENORRHOEA

This can be caused either by *cold* or by retardation of qi in the *gan-liver*. Invasion by the pathogen *cold* presents with pain during menstruation and a cold feeling in the lower abdomen which improves when the abdomen is warmed. There are dark red clots in the menses, the tongue coating is thin and white and the pulse deep and slow or bowstring. The qi in the *gan-liver* may be retarded by persistent depression or irritability. This presents with severe abdominal pain, distension in both flanks in the breasts and costal region. The menstrual fluid is purple with clots; the tongue coating is dark red with purple spots and the pulse is excessive, the bowstring. Use moxa over Ren4 if there is invasion of cold.

Point Selection

Ren4 frees the flow of qi in the channel and should be used for invasion by cold (with moxa).

Liv3 regulates the function of the gan-liver.

Sp6 frees the flow of qi through the channels in the genital region.

Shiquizhui (Extra) frees the channels.

Point Location

Sp6.   3 cun above the medial malleolus just posterior to the tibial border.

Liv3.   In the depression distal to the junction of the first and second metatarsal bones.

Ren4.   On the mid-line of the abdomen 3 cun below the umbilicus.

Shiquizhui. In the depression below the spinous process of the fifth lumbar vertebra on the mid-line between L5 and S1.

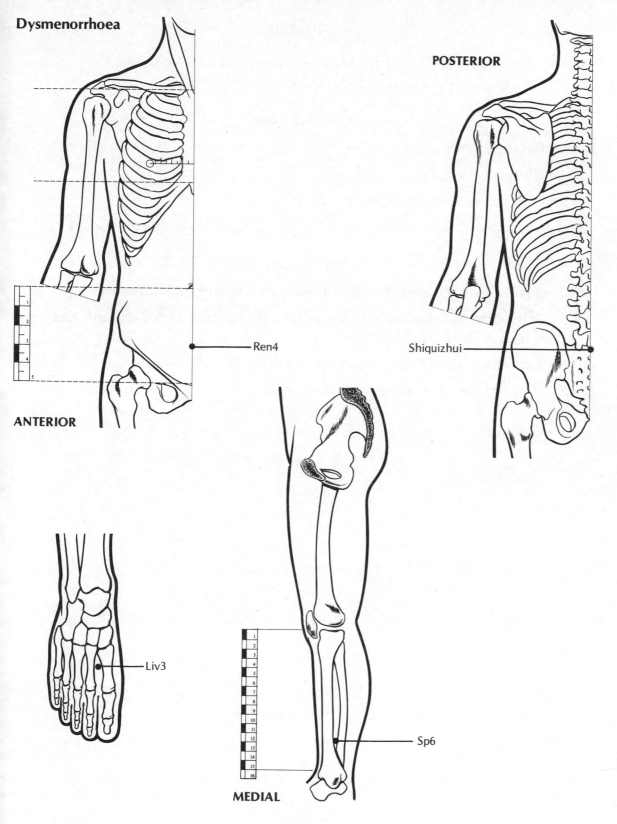

Dysmenorrhoea

POSTERIOR

Ren4

Shiquizhui

ANTERIOR

Liv3

Sp6

MEDIAL

83

ENURESIS

Enuresis is due to a deficiency of the *shen-kidney* and *pi-spleen*. This causes a lack of urinary control; treatment should be directed at the *shen-kidney* and *pi-spleen*.

Point Selection

K3 tonifies the kidney.

Sp6 tonifies and strengthens the pi-spleen.

Ren4 has direct local effect on the bladder.

Ren6 is the point of general tonification, and strengthens the body's resistance.

Point Location

Sp6.   3 cun above the medial malleolus just posterior to the tibial border.

K3.   In the depression between the medial malleolus and the tendo-calcaneus, level with the tip of the medial malleolus.

Ren4.   On the mid-line of the abdomen 3 cun below the umbilicus.

Ren6.   1.5 cun below the umbilicus in the mid-line.

Enuresis

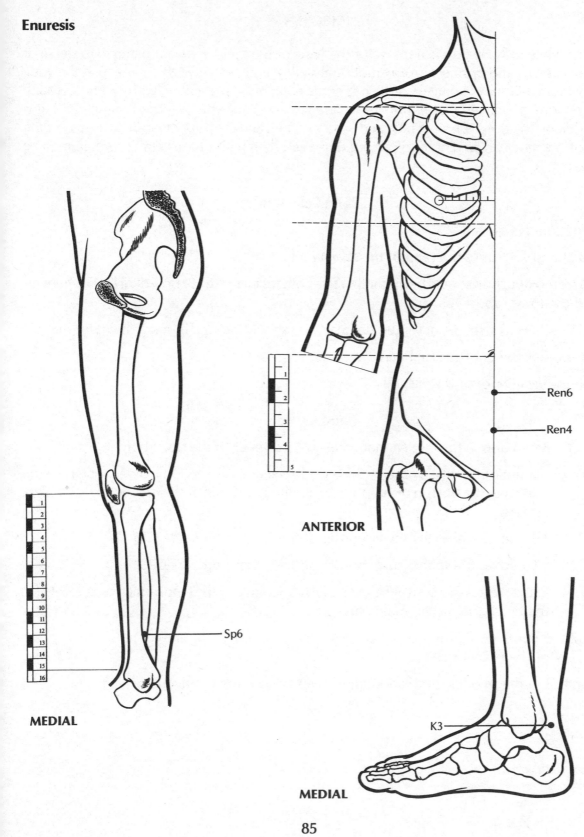

Ren6

Ren4

ANTERIOR

Sp6

MEDIAL

K3

MEDIAL

85

IMPOTENCE

Impotence may be due to damage of the yang of the *shen-kidney* or damage to the qi of the *xin-heart* and *pi-spleen* from emotional pathogens such as *fright* or *worry*. If the yang of the *shen-kidney* is damaged the patient is pale, often presenting with symptoms such as dizziness, blurred vision, urinary frequency and lumbar ache. The tongue coating is deficient, the tongue proper pale and tooth-marked and the pulse deep and thready. If the qi of the *xin-heart* and/or *pi-spleen* are damaged then palpitations and insomnia may be present.

Point Selection

Ren4 tonifies qi.

UB23 and K3 tonify the yang of the shen-kidney.

Du20, moxibustion should be applied to this point to increase the flow of qi in the channels and the lower abdomen.

UB15 is the back shu point for the xin-heart and should be used if the xin-heart is affected.

H7 tonifies the qi of the xin-heart.

Sp6 tonifies the qi of the pi-spleen.

Point Location

Sp6.   3 cun above the medial malleolus just posterior to the tibial border.

H7.   On the transverse crease of the wrist in the articular region between the pisiform bone and the ulna, in the depression on the radial side of the tendon of flexor carpi ulnaris.

UB15.   1.5 cun lateral to the lower border of the spinous process of T5.

UB23.   1.5 cun lateral to the lower border of the spinous process of L2.

K3.   In the depression between the medial malleolus and the tendo-calcaneus, level with the tip of the medial malleolus.

Du20.   7 cun above the posterior hairline on the mid-point of the line connecting the apexes of the two auricles.

Ren4.   On the mid-line of the abdomen, 3 cun below the umbilicus.

Impotence

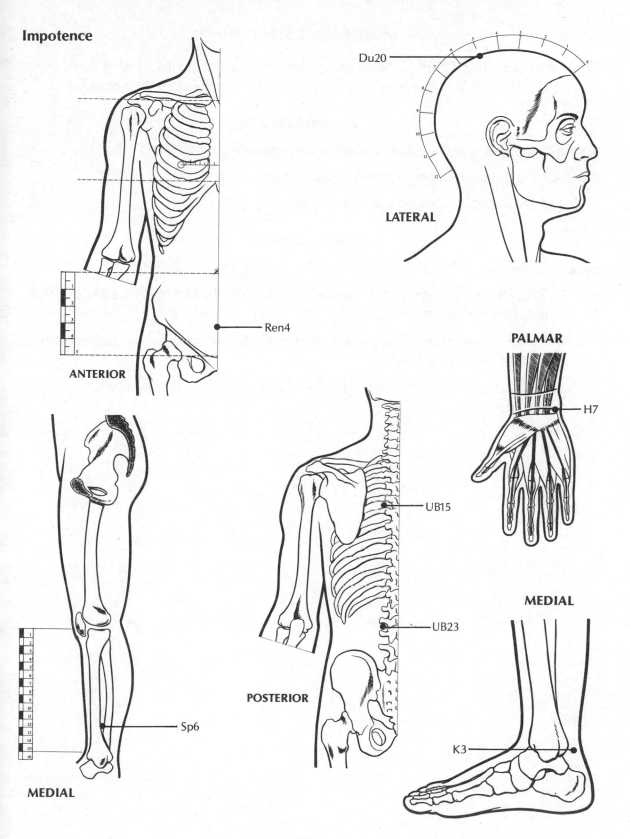

LATERAL

Du20

ANTERIOR

Ren4

PALMAR

H7

POSTERIOR

UB15

UB23

MEDIAL

MEDIAL

Sp6

K3

MENOPAUSAL SYMPTOMS

These symptoms result from a dysfunction of the *pi-spleen* and *gan-liver*. Tonify the *pi-spleen* and sedate the *gan-liver* (the liver and spleen channels run through the genitalia).

Point Selection

Sp6 and Sp4 stop vomiting, help dizziness and regulate the spleen.

P6 stops the adverse ascent of qi (vomiting and hot flushes).

Liv3 and P6 control palpitations and hot flushes.

Point Location

Sp6.   3 cun above the medial malleolus just posterior to the tibial border.

Sp4.   In the depression distal and inferior to the base of the first metatarsal bone, at the junction of the red and white skin.

P6.   2 cun above the transverse crease to the wrist between the tendons of palmaris longus and flexor carpi radialis.

Liv3.   In the depression distal to the junction of the first and second metatarsal bones.

Menopausal Symptoms

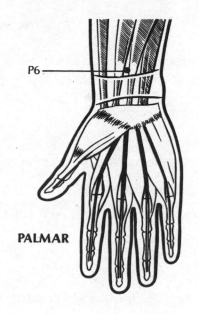

PALMAR

P6

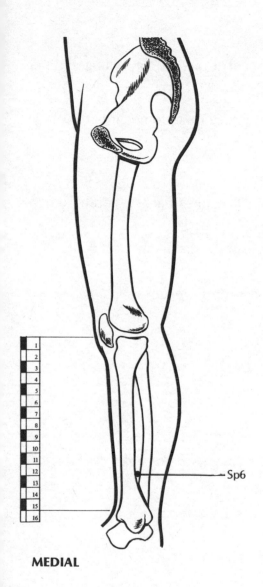

MEDIAL

Sp6

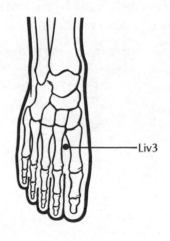

Liv3

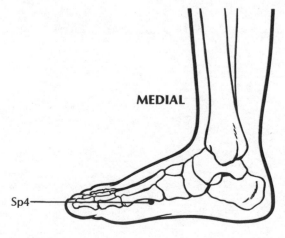

MEDIAL

Sp4

89

MORNING SICKNESS

During pregnancy qi and blood are directed to the Ren and Chong channels. This nourishes the baby but can lead to a lack of qi and blood in the rest of the mother's body. The *excess of qi in the Ren and Chong channels* can invade the stomach channel and cause vomiting.

Point Selection

P6 controls the middle jiao and stops the adverse ascent of qi, thereby controlling vomiting.

St36 regulates the stomach.

Sp4 connects with the Chong channels to regulate the pi-spleen and stomach (cardinal point for the Chong channel).

Point Location

St36. 3 cun below the lateral aspect of the knee joint line, one finger's breadth from the anterior crest to the tibia.

Sp4. In the depression distal and inferior to the base of the first metatarsal bone, at the junction of the red and white skin.

P6. 2 cun above the transverse crease to the wrist between the tendons of palmaris longus and flexor carpi radialis.

Morning Sickness

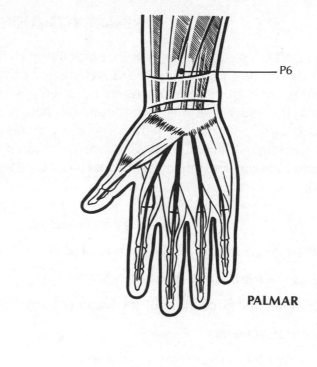

P6

PALMAR

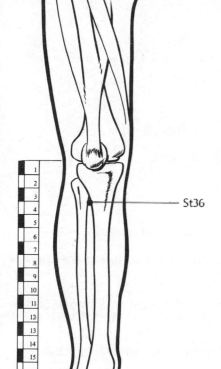

St36

ANTERIOR

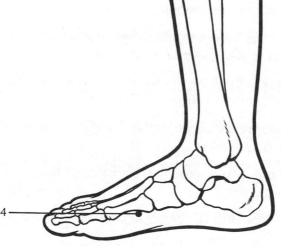

Sp4

MEDIAL

URINARY RETENTION

This can result from *surgical operations,* particularly on the lower abdomen, in which the channels themselves are damaged or insufficiency of yang of the *shen-kidney*. Surgical operations result in either complete retention or retention with overflow. There is distension and pain in the lower abdomen, the tongue has petechiae on it and the pulse is thready and rapid. Insufficiency of yang of the *shen-kidney* causes nocturia, dribbling and poor force in the urinary flow. The patient is weak and pale, often with a lumbar ache. The tongue has deficient coating and the tongue proper is pale and tooth-marked. The pulse is thready and weak.

Point Selection

Ren3 is the front mu point of the urinary bladder.

Sp6 adjusts the function of the urinary bladder.

UB39 promotes the circulation of the water passages.

1. **Surgical procedures**

Sp10 activates the channels and collaterals promoting the flow of qi in the damaged channels.

2. **Insufficiency of yang of the shen-kidney**

Du20. Apply moxa to this point, it activates the flow of qi in the bladder area.

Ren4 strengthens the qi of the shen-kidney to promote urination.

Point Location

Sp6. 3 cun above the medial malleolus just posterior to the tibial border.

Sp10. 2 cun above the mediosuperior border of the patella on the bulge of the medial portion of the quadriceps femoris.

UB39. In the popliteal crease, 1 cun lateral to the middle of the popliteal crease on the medial border of the biceps femoris.

Du20. 7 cun above the posterior hairline on the mid-point of the line connecting the apexes of the two oracles.

Ren3. 4 cun below the umbilicus and 1 cun above the border of the synthesis pubis, on the mid-line.

Ren4. On the mid-line of the abdomen 3 cun below the umbilicus.

Urinary Retention

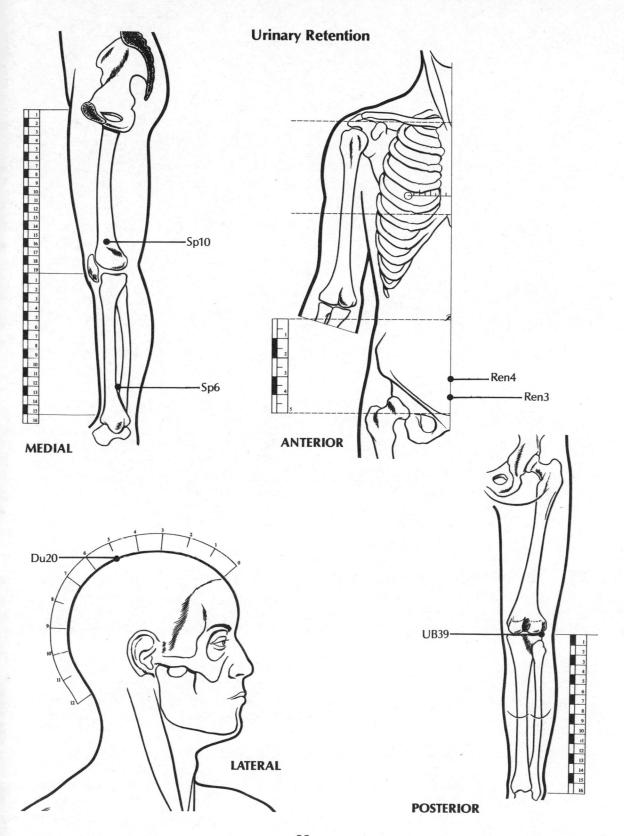

MEDIAL

Sp10

Sp6

ANTERIOR

Ren4

Ren3

Du20

LATERAL

UB39

POSTERIOR

93

11.

Psychological Problems

ANXIETY

The main organ that is disturbed in an anxiety state is the *xin-heart*. If the mental pathogen *fright* affects the *xin-heart* then a deficiency of qi and blood becomes apparent causing a mental disturbance. In an agitated state the *xin-heart* can be disturbed by endogenous *fire*. If the *xin-heart* fails to function properly then an inadequate circulation of the fluid results, this may cause palpitations varying from mild to uncontrollable.

If there is *insufficiency of qi and blood* the patient will present with pallor, dyspnoea, insomnia and blurred vision. The tongue will be pale, flabby and tooth-marked and the pulse deficient. If the patient presents with symptoms caused by endogenous *fire* then they will be irritable and restless. The tongue coating will be yellow and the pulse rapid and rolling. If the xin-heart is not functioning properly then the patient will have a cough with mucoid sputum, a full feeling in the chest and epigastrium and will complain of malaise. The tongue coating will be white with a rapid rolling pulse.

Point selection

The xin-heart is the main organ requiring treatment.

UB15 is the back shu point of the xin-heart.

H7 tonifies the xin-heart and is the yuan source point on the heart channel.

P6 strengthens the function of H7.

1. **Insufficiency of qi and blood**

Ren6 strengthens the qi.

UB20 adjusts the function of the pi-spleen which is always abnormal in insufficiency of qi and blood.

UB21 adjusts the function of the stomach and supports the action of UB20.

2. Endogenous fire

St40 disperses the pathogen phlegm, often associated with endogenous fire.

GB34 eliminates fire from the stomach.

3. Dysfunction of the xin-heart

Ren4, Ren17 and St36 work together to strengthen the function of the pi-spleen and invigorate the xin-heart and fei-lung, eliminating the production of harmful fluid.

UB22 regulates the function of the sanjiao (it is the back shu point for the sanjiao) and promotes the transportation of water.

Ren12 should be used if there is epigastric discomfort.

Point Location

St40. 8 cun superior and anterior to the lateral malleolus, two fingers' breadth lateral from the tibial crest.

H7. On the transverse crease of the wrist in the articular region between the pisiform bone and the ulna, in the depression on the radial side of the tendon of flexor carpi ulnaris.

UB15. 1.5 cun lateral to the lower border of the spinous process of T5.

UB20. 1.5 cun lateral to the lower border of the spinous process of T11.

UB21. 1.5 cun lateral to the lower border of the spinous process of T12.

UB22. 1.5 cun lateral to the lower border of the spinous process of L1.

P6. 2 cun above the transverse crease to the wrist between the tendons of palmaris longus and flexor carpi radialis.

GB34. In the depression anterior and inferior to the head of the fibula.

Ren6. 1.5 cun below the umbilicus in the mid-line.

Ren12. On the mid-line of the abdomen between the navel and the xiphisternum, 4 cun above the umbilicus.

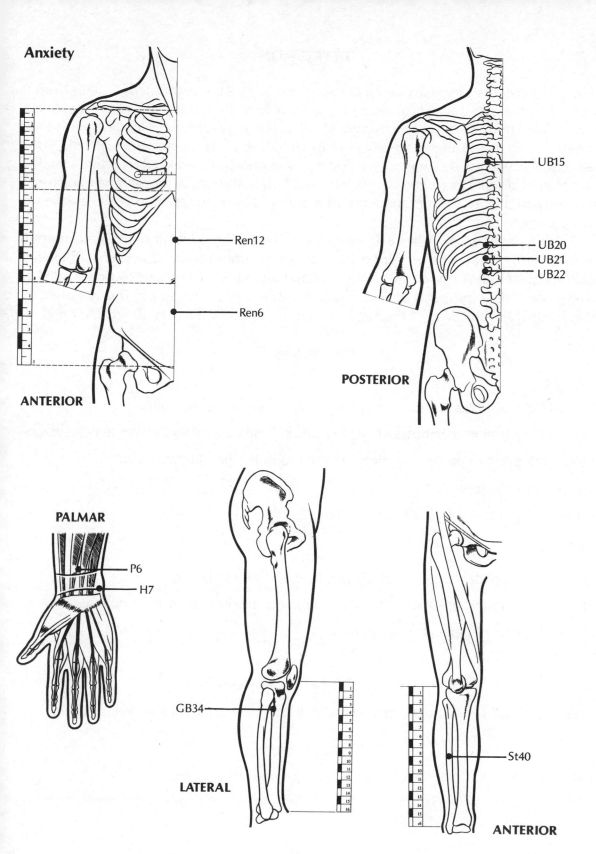

Anxiety

ANTERIOR

Ren12

Ren6

POSTERIOR

UB15

UB20
UB21
UB22

PALMAR

P6

H7

LATERAL

GB34

ANTERIOR

St40

97

DEPRESSION

This may be caused by injury to the *pi-spleen, xin-heart, gan-liver* or *shen-kidney. Overjoy, fear or fright* affects the *xin-heart,* excessive *anger* affects the *gan-liver* and excessive *anxiety, grief or over-thinking* (including overwork) will affect the *pi-spleen.* A long chronic illness drains the yin qi and affects the *shen-kidney.* Xu depression presents with insomnia, sleep disturbance, vertigo, poor memory, palpitations, anorexia, malaise and sometimes tinnitus and blurred vision. The tongue coating is thin and white, the tongue proper is pale and tooth-marked and the pulse is soft, thready and forceless. The main organs affected are the *xin-heart, pi-spleen* and *shen-kidney.*

A shi depression is more like a depressive illness associated with anxiety. The symptoms include vertigo, headache, a feeling of fullness or distension in the head, insomnia, irritability, pain and distension in the costal and hypochondriac region. The tongue coating is thin and white, the tongue proper is red and the pulse thready but bowstring. This is caused by hyperactivity of the yang of the gan-liver and an excess of fire that affects the mind.

Point Selection

Xu type

P6 and H7 work together to calm the mind and soothe the mentality.

Yintang (Extra) reinforces the function of P6 and H7 and is useful for the symptom headache.

St36 is the point of general tonification and promotes the function of Sp6.

Sp6 tonifies the pi-spleen.

K3 and K7 nourish the yin of the shen-kidney.

Shi type

Liv3 and Liv4 pacify the yang of the gan-liver and tonify the yin.

Sp6 and Sp9 tonify the pi-spleen and promote the absorption of nourishing qi.

LI4 is the point of general tonification.

SJ6 resolves depression.

GB20 is a useful symptomatic point for headache and vertigo.

Ren12 is useful for epigastric discomfort; it is the influential point of the fu organs.

Point Location

LI4.   In the middle of the first metacarpal on the radial aspect.

St36.   3 cun below the lateral aspect of the knee joint line, one finger's breadth from the anterior crest of the tibia.

Depression

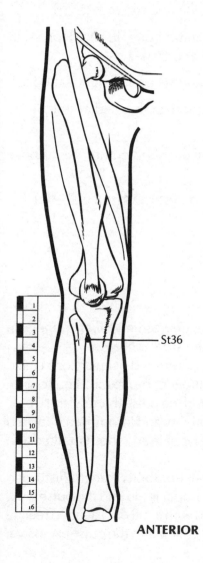

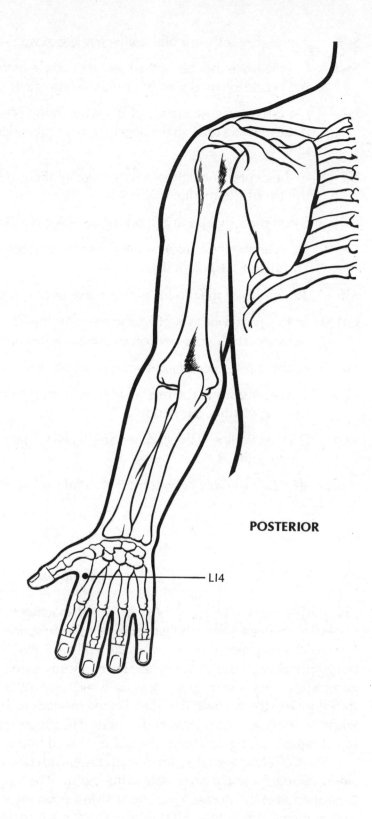

St36

ANTERIOR

POSTERIOR

LI4

Sp6.   3 cun above the medial malleolus just posterior to the tibial border.

Sp9.   On the lower border of the medial condyle of the tibia, in the depression between the posterior border of the tibia and the gastrocnemius.

H7.   On the transverse crease of the wrist in the articular region between the pisiform bone and the ulna, in the depression on the radial side of the tendon of flexor carpi ulnaris.

K3.   In the depression between the medial malleolus and the tendo-calcaneus, level with the tip of the medial malleolus.

K7.   2 cun directly above K3, on the anterior border of the tendo-calcaneus.

P6.   2 cun above the transverse crease to the wrist between the tendons of palmaris longus and flexor carpi radialis.

SJ6.   3 cun above the medial wrist crease between the ulna and the radius.

GB20. In the posterior aspect of the neck, below the occipital bone, in the depression between the upper portion of sternocleidomastoid and trapezius.

Liv3. In the depression distal to the junction of the first and second metatarsal bones.

Liv4. 1 cun anterior to the medial malleolus in the depression on the medial side of the tendon of tibialis anterior.

Ren12. On the mid-line of the abdomen between the navel and the xiphisternum, 4 cun above the umbilicus.

Yintang (Extra). Midway between the medial end of the two eyebrows (the glabella).

INSOMNIA

This can be caused by xu of the *pi-spleen,* disharmony of the *xin-heart* and *shen-kidney,* an excess of the yang qi of the *gan-liver* or a dysfunction of the *stomach.*
Xu of the *pi-spleen* presents with a difficulty in falling asleep, disturbed sleep accompanied by palpitations, poor memory, malaise, anorexia and a sallow complexion. The tongue coating is greasy, the tongue proper pale and tooth-marked and the pulse thready and weak. Imbalance in the *xin-heart* and *shen-kidney* presents with irritability and insomnia associated with dizziness, low back pain and tinnitus. The tongue proper is pale and tooth-marked and the tongue coating deficient, the pulse is rapid and weak.
Excess of yang qi of the *gan-liver* presents with depression, irritability, dream disturbed sleep, headache and a bitter taste in the mouth. The tongue proper is red and the pulse wiry. Dysfunction of the *stomach* presents with insomnia associated with a full or distended feeling in the epigastric region and flatulence. The tongue coating is greasy and the pulse excessive.

Depression

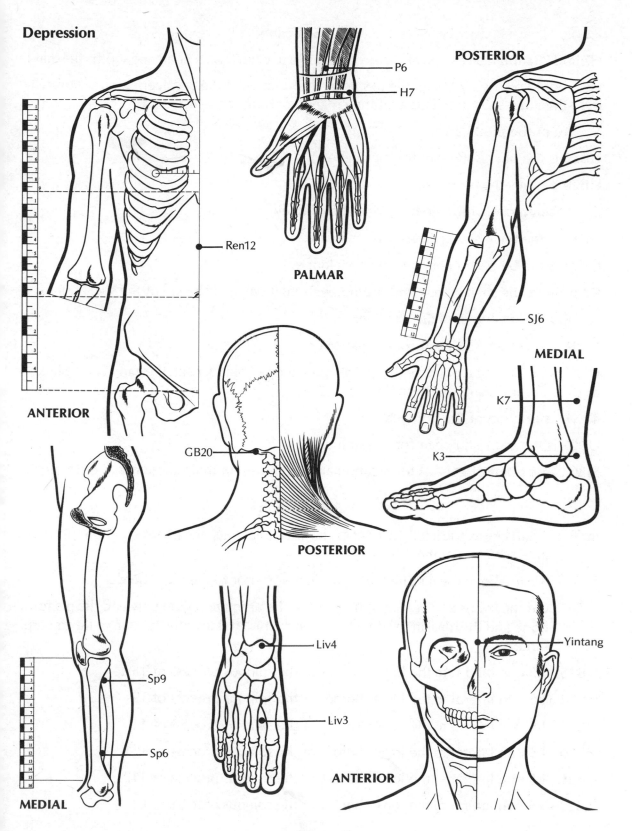

ANTERIOR

Ren12

PALMAR

P6

H7

POSTERIOR

SJ6

MEDIAL

K7

K3

GB20

POSTERIOR

MEDIAL

Sp9

Sp6

Liv4

Liv3

ANTERIOR

Yintang

101

Point Selection

H7 and P6 should be used in all cases of insomnia to calm the xin-heart and soothe the mind.

Sp6 should be used to tonify the pi-spleen; dysfunction of the pi-spleen can be caused by over-thinking, a common precipitating mental pathogen for insomnia.

1. Xu of the pi-spleen

UB15 is the back shu point for the xin-heart.

UB20 tonifies the pi-spleen.

2. Disharmony of the xin-heart and shen-kidney

UB15 is the back shu point for the xin-heart.

UB23 is the back shu point for the shen-kidney.

K3 tonifies the shen-kidney and promotes strengthening of the yin of the shen-kidney.

3. Excess of yang qi of the gan-liver

UB18 is the back shu point for the gan-liver.

UB19 is the back shu point for the gall bladder (the gall bladder and the gan-liver are linked both structurally and functionally).

4. Dysfunction of the stomach

UB21 is the back shu point for the stomach.

St36 is the point of general tonification and promotes normal function in the stomach.

Point Location

St36. 3 cun below the lateral aspect of the knee joint line, one finger's breadth from the anterior crest of the ibia.

Sp6. 3 cun above the medial malleolus just posterior to the tibial border.

H7. On the transverse crease of the wrist in the articular region between the pisiform bone and the ulna, in the depression on the radial side of the tendon of flexor carpi ulnaris.

UB15. 1.5 cun lateral to the lower border of the spinous process of T5.

UB18. 1.5 cun lateral to the lower border of the spinous process of T9.

UB19. 1.5 cun lateral to the lower border of the spinous process of T10.

UB20. 1.5 cun lateral to the lower border of the spinous process of T11.

UB21. 1.5 cun lateral to the lower border of the spinous process of T12.

UB23. 1.5 cun lateral to the lower border of the spinous process of L2.

Insomnia

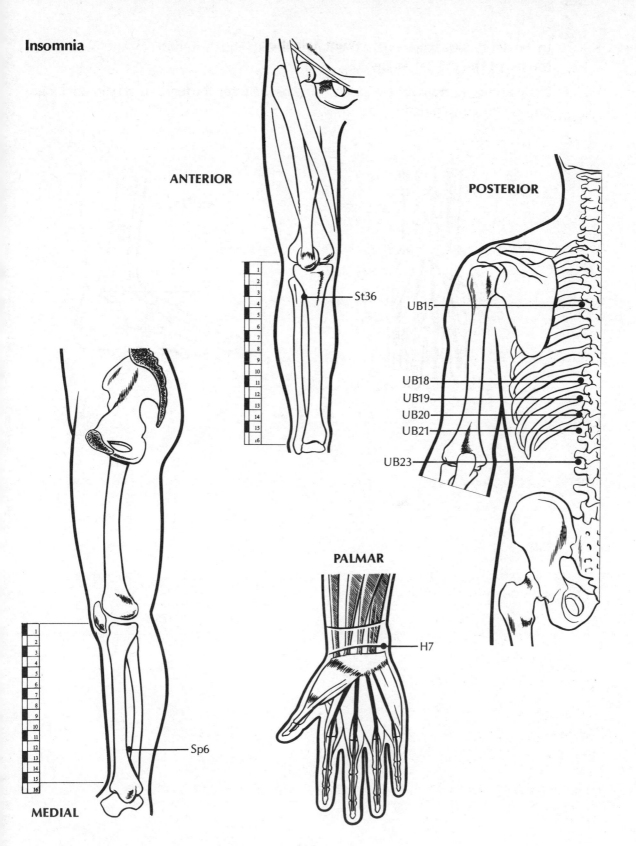

ANTERIOR

St36

POSTERIOR

UB15

UB18
UB19
UB20
UB21

UB23

MEDIAL

Sp6

PALMAR

H7

K3.   In the depression between the medial malleolus and the tendo-calcaneus, level with the tip of the medial malleolus.

P6.   2 cun above the transverse crease to the wrist between the tendons of palmaris longus and flexor carpi radialis.

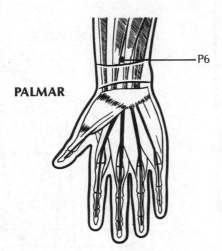

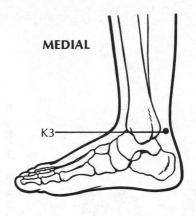

12.

Neurological Conditions

FACIAL NERVE PARALYSIS

This is caused by the invasion of the pathogens *wind* and *cold,* which results in an obstruction of the free flow of qi and blood. The patient presents with impaired facial movement on the affected side, there may also be pain behind the root of the ear. The tongue coating is thin and white and the pulse floating and tight.

Choose points on the face where the paralysis seems to have maximum effect; the points from the large intestine and stomach channels are particularly useful for the treatment of this condition. Needles should be inserted and needling sensation obtained, but electrical stimulation is of great value in treating this condition.

Point Selection

SJ17 has a strong action in removing obstructions and dispelling wind; it is also particularly useful for alleviating any pain that may be associated with the facial paralysis. Puncture deeply.

GB14, Taiyang (Extra) and SI18 are all situated on the respective divisions of the seventh nerve. They free and invigorate qi and blood in the local areas.

St4 and St6 are particularly useful in removing local obstructions to the channels.

LI4 is the distal point of the large intestine channel and useful in dispersing wind.

Liv3 disperses internal wind.

SI18. Patients with chronic facial paralysis will benefit from cupping on this point.

Point Location

LI4.   In the middle of the first metacarpal on the radial aspect.

St4.   On the corner of the mouth, directly below the middle of the eyebrow.

St6.   One finger's breadth anterior and superior to the lower angle of the mandible, where masseter attaches at the prominence of the muscle when the teeth are clenched.

SI18.   Directly below the outer canthus of the eye in the depression below the lower border of the zygomatic bone.

SJ17.   Posterior to the lobule of the ear in the depression between the mandible and mastoid process.

GB14.   On the forehead, 1 cun above the mid-point of the eyebrow.

Liv3.   In the depression distal to the junction of the first and second metatarsal bones.

Taiyang (Extra). In the depression 1 cun posterior to the mid-point between the lateral end of the eyebrow and the outer canthus of the eye.

HEADACHE (including Migraine)

Headaches may be due to hyperactivity of the yang of the *gan-liver, xu* or deficiency of *blood* and invasion of the *pi-spleen* by *phlegm* and *damp*. Exogenous factors such as *wind and heat* or *wind and cold* may also cause headaches; these are often associated with acute viral infections.

Hyperactivity of the *gan-liver* presents with dizziness, irritability, a flushed face and a pounding headache (migraine). Visual disturbances often occur prior to the headache and there is usually some photophobia during the headache. The tongue coating is thin and yellow and the pulse is bowstring. Headaches caused by a deficiency of blood (xu) present with lassitude, palpitations, pallor and a dull continuous headache. The tongue coating is thin and white, the tongue proper white and tooth-marked and the pulse is deficient. When *phlegm* and *damp* invade the *pi-spleen* the patient is often obese and tends to over-indulge in food. They present with a feeling of fullness and distension in the chest, abdomen and head associated with nausea and/or vomiting. The tongue coating is thin, white and greasy and the pulse gliding.

Facial Nerve Paralysis

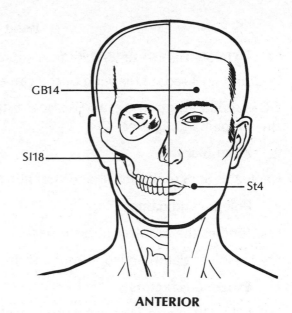

ANTERIOR

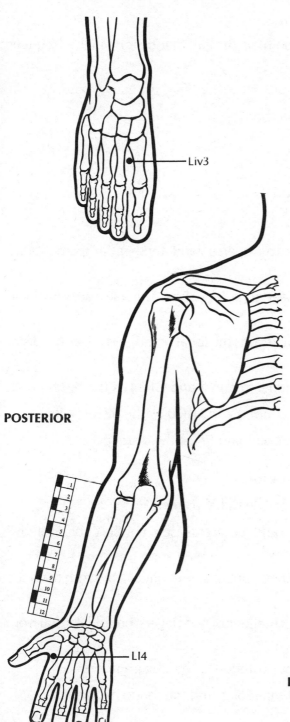

POSTERIOR

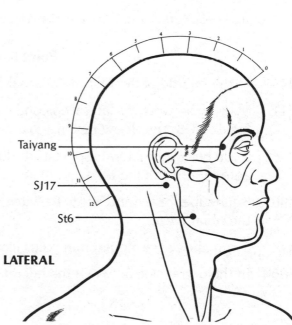

LATERAL

Point Selection

1. Hyperactivity of the gan-liver

Liv3 and Liv8 sedate the yang of the gan-liver.

GB34 sedates the gan-liver and is also a distal point on the gall-bladder channel, a frequent site for pain in migraine.

2. Xu of blood

Ren6 and St36 tonify the qi and strengthen the body.

3. Phlegm and damp

Sp6 tonifies the pi-spleen and stomach.

St40 resolves damp and tonifies the stomach.

4. Exogenous factors

LI4, LI11, Du14 and SJ5 can be used together to disperse wind and heat and ameliorate headaches caused by acute viral infections.

Points should be used according to the site of headache, they should be selected using local and distal points.

For a *frontal headache,* use GB14 and Yintang (Extra) as the local points and LI4 as the distal point.

For *migraine* use tender points on the gall-bladder channel and GB34 as the distal point.

For *occipital headaches,* use GB20 as the local point and UB60 as the distal point.

For *vertical headaches,* use Du20 as the local point and P6 as the distal point.

Point Location

LI4. In the middle of the first metacarpal on the radial aspect.

LI11. Midway between the lateral epicondyle and the lateral aspect of the cubital (elbow) crease, with the elbow flexed.

St36. 3 cun below the lateral aspect of the knee joint line, one finger's breadth from the anterior crest of the tibia.

St40. 8 cun superior and anterior to the lateral malleolus, two fingers' breadth lateral from the tibial crest.

Sp6. 3 cun above the medial malleolus just posterior to the tibial border.

UB60. In the depression between the lateral malleolus and the tendo-calcaneus.

Headache

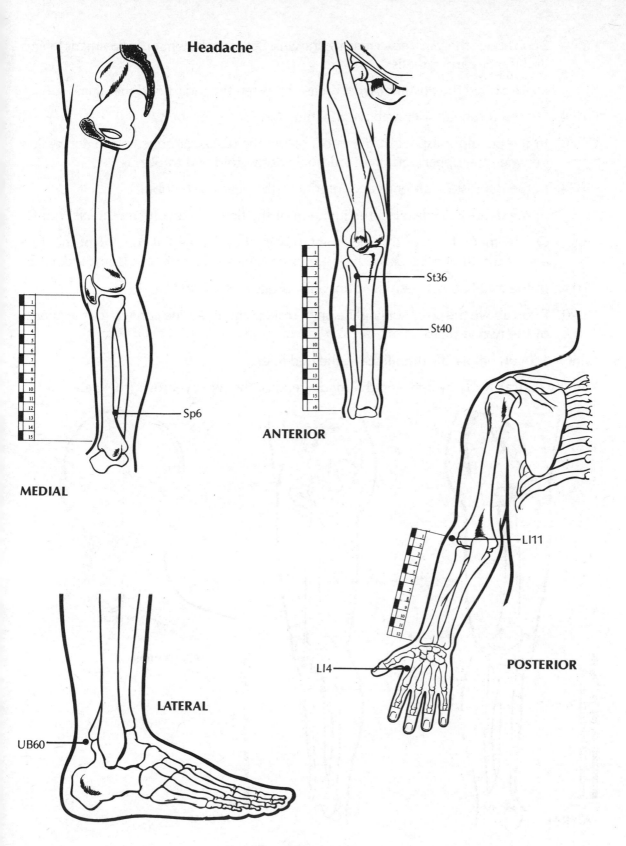

MEDIAL

Sp6

ANTERIOR

St36

St40

POSTERIOR

LI11

LI4

LATERAL

UB60

P6. 2 cun above the transverse crease to the wrist between the tendons of palmaris longus and flexor carpi radialis.

SJ5. 2 cun above the posterior wrist crease between the radius and the ulna.

GB14. On the forehead, 1 cun above the mid-point of the eyebrow.

GB20. In the posterior aspect of the neck, below the occipital bone, in the depression between the upper portion of sternocleidomastoid and trapezius.

GB34. In the depression anterior and inferior to the head of the fibula.

Liv3. In the depression distal to the junction of the first and second metatarsal bones.

Liv8. On the medial side of the knee joint, posterior to the medial condyle of the tibia and on the anterior border of the insertion of semimembranosus and semitendinosus.

Du14. In the mid-line between the transverse process of C7 and T1.

Du20. 7 cun above the posterior hairline on the mid-point of the line connecting the apexes of the two auricles.

Ren6. 1.5 cun below the umbilicus in the mid-line.

Yintang (Extra). Midway between the medial end of the two eyebrows (the glabella).

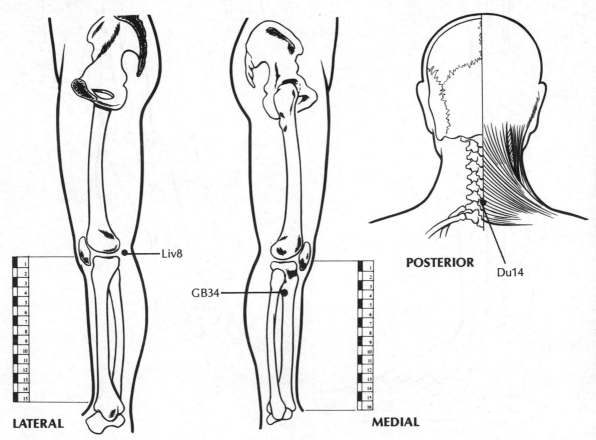

LATERAL   MEDIAL

110

Headache

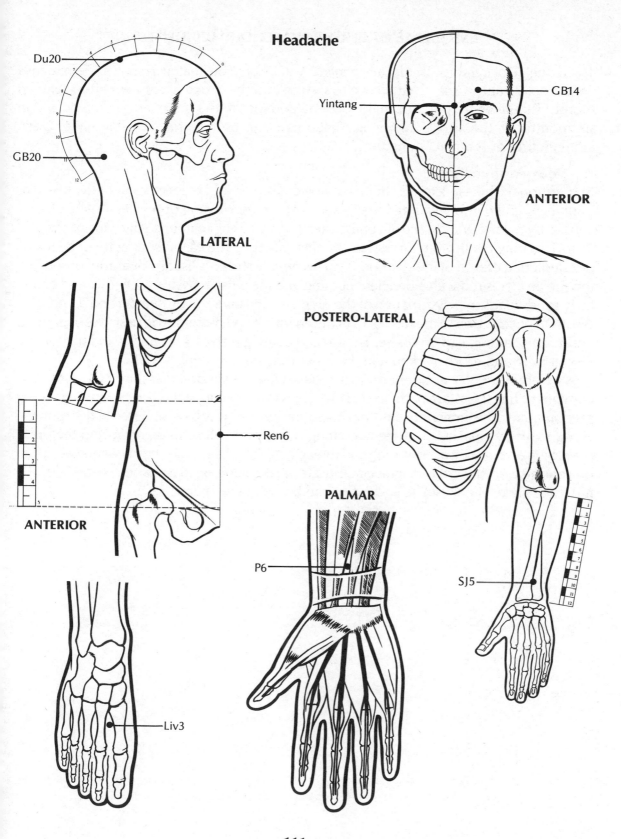

Du20

GB20

LATERAL

Yintang

GB14

ANTERIOR

POSTERO-LATERAL

Ren6

ANTERIOR

PALMAR

P6

SJ5

Liv3

111

SEQUELAE OF CEREBROVASCULAR ACCIDENTS

The sequelae of cerebrovascular accidents (C.V.A.) should be treated as soon as the patient's condition is stable, usually within two to six weeks of the stroke. Treatment after eighteen months is unlikely to produce major benefit, and ideally the treatment should be within six months of the stroke occurring. Treatment can be directed at using either body acupuncture or scalp acupuncture.

1.   Body Acupuncture

In traditional Chinese terms a stroke may be caused by an excess of yang of the *gan-liver* or *phlegm* and *damp* invading the *pi-spleen*. An excess of yang of the *gan-liver* is usually caused by a deficiency of the yin of the *shen-kidney* failing to nourish the yang of the *gan-liver*. This may result from an excess of *anger* affecting the *gan-liver* directly or a lack of rest depleting the yin of the *shen-kidney*. This type of stroke is usually of abrupt onset. The tongue proper is red with a deficient coating and the pulse bowstring. Obesity and eating fatty foods leads to a dysfunction of the *pi-spleen* and invasion by *phlegm* and *damp*. This results in obstruction to the flow of qi in the channels and presents with a stroke of gradual onset. The patient is often obese. The tongue coating is thick and greasy and the tongue proper pale and tooth-marked and the pulse may be bowstring or deficient.

A cerebrovascular accident may also be divided in shi or xu. A shi C.V.A. is often a combination of the above pathological processes in their acute stage, one type usually being predominant. The illness is usually of short duration and may be associated with dizziness, vertigo and dysphasia. The tongue coating is thin and yellow and greasy and the pulse bowstring and gliding or bowstring and thready. Xu C.V.A.s are the chronic sequelae, often presenting with flaccid hemiphlegia, muscle wasting and/or spasm and spasticity of the muscles. There is an insufficiency of qi and blood in the channels.

Point Selection

1. Excess of yang

LI4 tonifies qi.

Liv3 pacifies the gan-liver and eliminates wind.

UB18 is the back shu point for the gan-liver.

K3 regulates the shen-kidney, reinforcing its yin.

GB34 eliminates the wind of the gan-liver.

2. Excess of phlegm and damp

LI4 tonifies qi.

SJ5 regulates the middle jiao and removes damp.

Sp6 tonifies the pi-spleen.

St40 resolves damp.

UB20 is the back shu point for the pi-spleen.

3. Shi type

This is usually a combination of the above two pathological processes and points should be chosen from the above prescriptions.

4. Xu type

It is important to tonify the circulation of qi and blood in the main channels of the body. Therefore select commonly used points on the major muscle groups and/or limbs that are affected by the stroke.

5. Points according to symptoms

Points may be selected according to specific symptoms, these are:
a) Facial paralysis (see page 105).

b) Aphasia and a stiff tongue, Ren23, K6, H5.

c) Spasticity in the arm, Lu5, P6 and H3.

d) Spasticity in the leg, Sp6, K3 and St41.

e) For shoulder pain, SJ14 and LI15.

f) For hip pain, GB29 and St31.

Point Location

Lu5. On the cubital crease, on the radial side of the biceps tendon.

LI4. In the middle of the first metacarpal on the radial aspect.

LI15. Antero inferior to the acromion, in the middle of the upper portion of the deltoid.

St31. Directly below the anterior superior iliac spine in the depression on the lateral side of the sartorius, when the thigh is flexed.

St40. 8 cun superior and anterior to the lateral malleolus, two fingers' breadth lateral from the tibial crest.

St41. At the junction of the dorsum of the foot and the leg between the tendons of extensor digitorum longus and hallucis longus.

Sp6. 3 cun above the medial malleolus just posterior to the tibial border.

H3. When the elbow is flexed this point is at the medial end of the transverse cubital crease, in the depression anterior to the medial epicondyle of the humerus.

H5. When the palm faces upwards this point is on the radial side of the tendon of the flexor carpi ulnaris, 1 cun above the transverse wrist crease.

UB18. 1.5 cun lateral to the lower border of the spinous process of T9.

UB20. 1.5 cun lateral to the lower border of the spinous process of T11.

K3. In the depression between the medial malleolus and the tendo-calcaneus, level with the tip of the medial malleolus.

K6. 1 cun below the medial malleolus.

P6. 2 cun above the transverse crease to the wrist between the tendons of palmaris longus and flexor carpi radialis.

SJ5. 2 cun above the posterior wrist crease between the radius and the ulna.

SJ14. Posterior and inferior to the acromion, 1 cun posterior to LI15.

GB29. Midway between the anterior superior iliac spine and the greater trochanter.

GB34. In the depression anterior and inferior to the head of the fibula.

Liv3. In the depression distal to the junction of the first and second metatarsal bones.

Ren23. Above the Adam's apple in the depression at the upper border of the hyoid bone.

Note:
Needling sensation should be sought on each needle inserted, although it may not always be possible to obtain deqi if the patient is suffering from a stroke. Ideally local points should be stimulated electrically, this is particularly useful in overcoming spasticity.

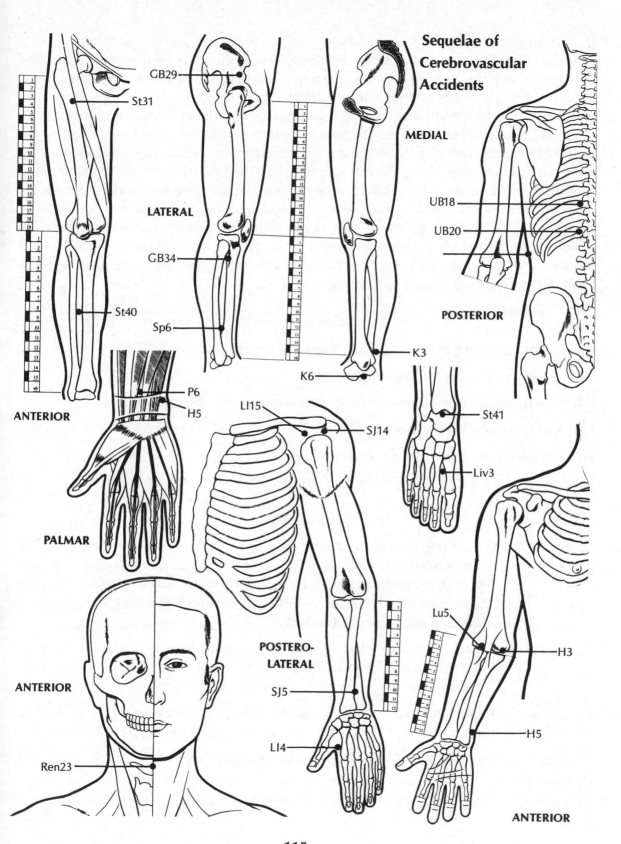

Sequelae of
Cerebrovascular
Accidents

GB29

St31

MEDIAL

LATERAL

GB34

Sp6

St40

ANTERIOR

UB18

UB20

POSTERIOR

K3

K6

P6

H5

LI15

SJ14

St41

Liv3

PALMAR

Lu5

H3

POSTERO-
LATERAL

ANTERIOR

SJ5

H5

LI4

Ren23

ANTERIOR

115

II.   Scalp Acupuncture

Scalp acupuncture is probably better than body acupuncture for the treatment of strokes. The principle of this therapy is simple, the aim being to stimulate the diseased area of the brain in order to facilitate a return of function in that area. The method is based on elementary functional neuro-anatomy and has nothing to do with traditional Chinese medicine. If part of the brain is damaged then the scalp should be stimulated over the area representing the impaired function; the scalp should be stimulated bilaterally and electro-stimulation should be used on the needles, using a high frequency (1,000 hertz) for at least thirty minutes and preferably one hour at each consultation. Scalp acupuncture probably works by increasing local vascularity and should therefore not be used until the stroke has been stable for at least two weeks. The Chinese often insert long needles (two- or three-inches) along the scalp region, between the dermis and periosteum. It is often easier, and less painful, for the patient to insert a series of one-inch needles obliquely, stimulating the one at the top and at the base of the scalp area requiring treatment.

Point Selection

Use motor region for motor impairment and motor aphasia.

Use sensory region for sensory impairment.

Use foot motor sensory region for functional impairment of the lower limb.

Use speech region 2 for sensory aphasia.

Use speech region 3 for nominal aphasia.

Use vertigo region for hearing and balance problems.

Point Location

Motor area.   0.5 cm posterior to the midpoint of the anterior-posterior line defines the upper limit of the motor area. The lower limit intersects the eyebrow-occiput line at the anterior border of the natural hairline on the temple. The upper 1/5 represents the lower limbs and trunk, the middle 2/5 represents the upper limbs and the lower 2/5 the face.

Sensory area.   This is a line parallel to the motor area and 1.5 cm behind it. The sensory input to the lower limbs and trunk is represented on the upper 1/5, the middle 2/5 represents the upper limbs, and the lower 2/5 represents the face.

Foot motor-sensory area.   Parallel to and 1 cm lateral to the anterior-posterior line. The line is 3 cm long and starts 1 cm posterior to the line representing the sensory area.

Chorea-tremor area.   Parallel to and 1.5 cm in front of the motor area.

Vasomotor area.   Parallel to and 1.5 cm in front of the chorea-tremor area.

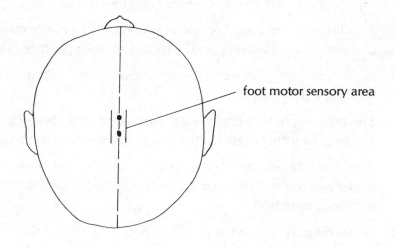

foot motor sensory area

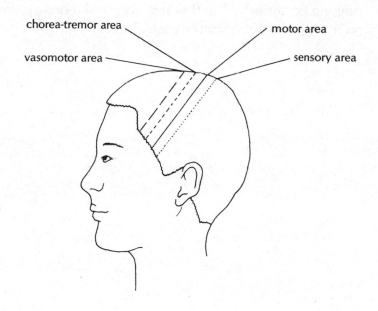

chorea-tremor area

motor area

vasomotor area

sensory area

Vertigo-auditory area.	A 4 cm horizontal line with its centre located 1.5 cm above the apex of the pinna.
First Speech or usage area.	Taking the parietal tubercule as a reference point insert three needles separately at 40° to each other. Each line is 3 cm long.
Second Speech area.	This line is 3 cm long and starts on a point 2 cm posterior-inferior to the parietal tubercule and parallel to the anterior-posterior line.
Third Speech area.	A 4 cm line originating at the mid-point of the vertigo-auditory area and running posteriorly.
Optic area.	This area originates 1 cm lateral to the mid-point of the occipital protuberance and runs for 4 cm parallel to the anterior-posterior line in an anterior direction.
Balance area.	This area originates 3 cm lateral to the mid-point of the occipital protuberance and runs for 4 cm parallel to the anterior-posterior line in a posterior direction.
Gastric area.	A line directly above the pupil starting from the hairline and running for 2 cm in a posterior direction parallel to the anterior-posterior line.
Thoracic area.	Midway between the anterior-posterior midline and the gastric area. It is a 4 cm line with its mid-point on the hairline, running parallel to the gastric area.
Reproduction area.	A 2 cm line paralleled to the gastric area originating at the hair line and running posteriorly. The thoracic area and reproduction area originate at points equidistant from the gastric area.

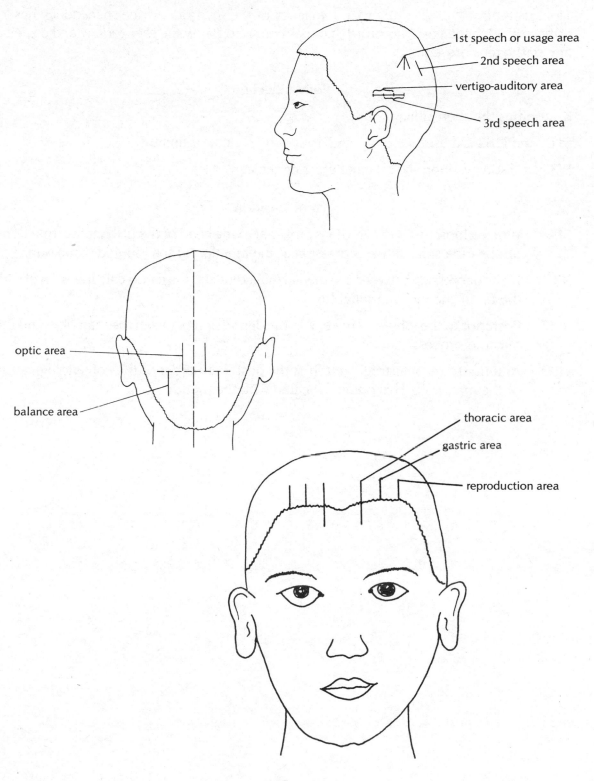

TINNITUS

Tinnitus is almost always due to a deficiency of the *shen-kidney* (the shen-kidney has its orifice through the ear). Therefore the treatment is to tonify the *shen-kidney* and disperse any pathogens present.

Point Selection

K3 tonifies the shen-kidney.

SJ17 and GB2 are useful local points for the treatment of tinnitus.

SI3 is a distal point on the channel crossing the ear.

Point Location

SI3.   When a loose fist is made, SI3 is proximal to the head of the fifth metacarpal bone on the ulna side, in the depression at the junction of the red and white skin.

K3.   In the depression between the medial malleolus and the tendo-calcaneus, level with the tip of the medial malleolus.

SJ17.   Posterior to the lobule of the ear, in the depression between the mandible and the mastoid process.

GB2.   Anterior to the intertragic notch at the posterior border of the condyloid process of the mandible. This point is located with the mouth open.

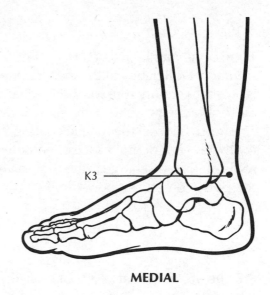

MEDIAL

POSTERIOR

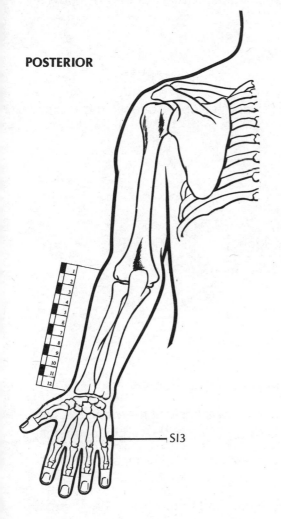

SI3

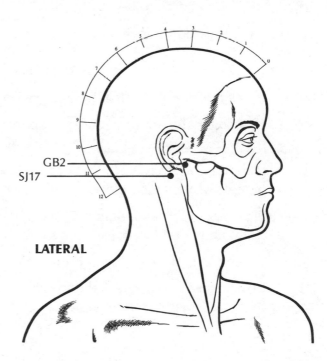

GB2

SJ17

LATERAL

121

TOOTHACHE

Toothache can be caused by a deficiency of the *shen-kidney* or excess of *fire from the stomach*. Deficiency of the *shen-kidney* causes a xu type toothache; if a xu type toothache is present acupuncture will only palliate the pain and dental advice must be sought swiftly. Xu toothache presents with vague intermittent pain, lassitude, and often a lumbar ache. The tooth is loose, the tongue coating thin and white and the pulse markedly deficient. Shi toothache is a dental abscess, and presents with continuous painful toothache, pus or a foul-smelling discharge in the mouth and fever. The tongue coating is thin and yellow and the pulse forceful or bowstring.

Point Selection

Shi type

St7 and St6 and local points of pain; they remove fire and the obstruction in the channels.

LI4 is a distal point for aching in the upper jaw.

St44 is a distal point for aching in the lower jaw.

Xu type

K3 tonifies the shen-kidney.

UB23 is the back shu point for tonifying the shen-kidney.

Distal points should be used as indicated above (LI4, St44).

GB20 should be added for headache.

SJ5 should be added for fever.

Point Location

LI4.   In the middle of the first metacarpal on the radial aspect.

St6.   One finger's breadth anterior and superior to the lower angle of the mandible, where masseter attaches at the prominence of the muscle when the teeth are clenched.

St7.   In the depression of the lower border of the zygomatic arch, anterior to the condyloid process of the mandible.

St44.   Proximal to the web margin between the second and third toes in the depression distal and lateral to the second metatarso digital joint.

UB23.   1.5 cun lateral to the lower border of the spinous process of L2.

K3.   In the depression between the medial malleolus and the tendo-calcaneus, level with the tip of the medial malleolus.

Toothache

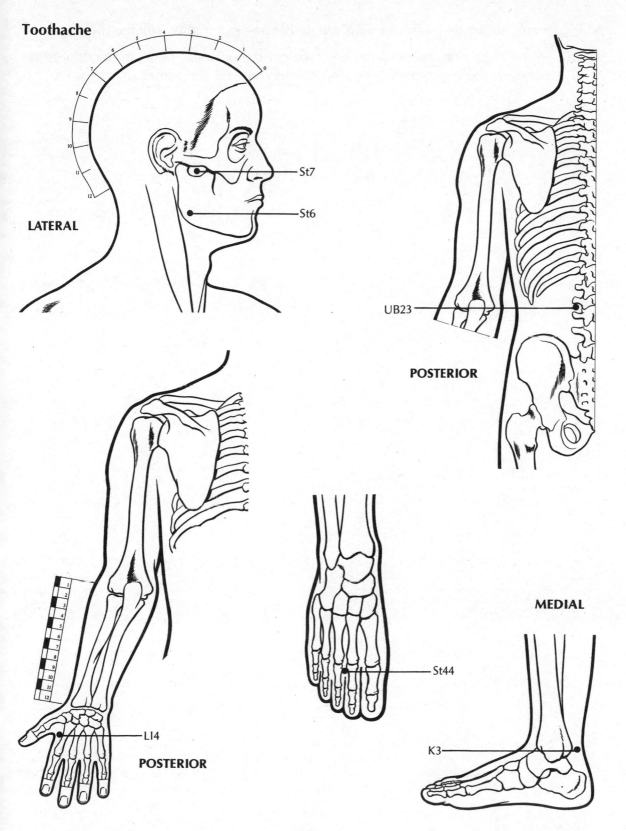

LATERAL

St7

St6

POSTERIOR

UB23

POSTERIOR

LI4

St44

MEDIAL

K3

123

SJ5.   2 cun above the posterior wrist crease between the radius and the ulna.

GB20. In the posterior aspect of the neck, below the occipital bone, in the depression between the upper portion of sternocleidomastoid and trapezius.

Toothache

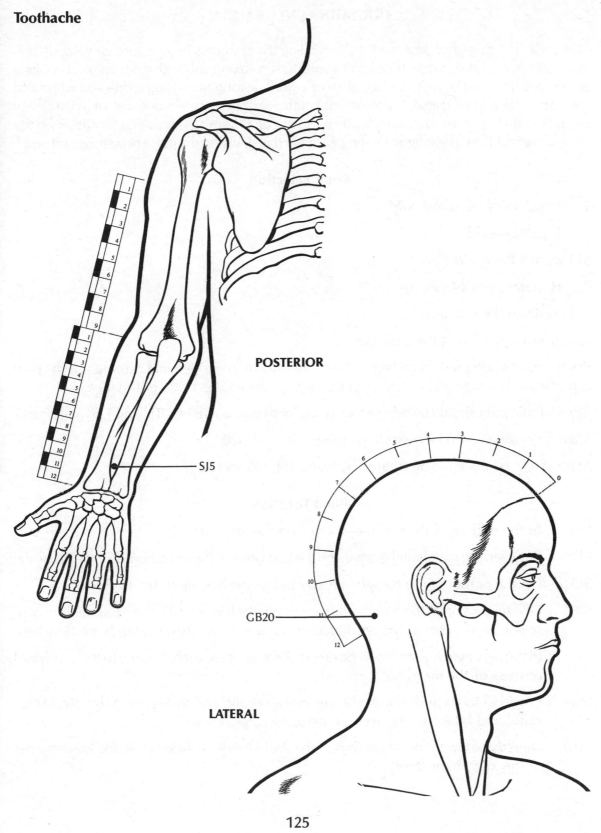

POSTERIOR

SJ5

GB20

LATERAL

125

TRIGEMINAL NEURALGIA

This is caused by either *wind* and *cold* invading the channels or an excess of yang qi (fire) in the *gan-liver* and *stomach*. Invasion by wind and cold presents with a paroxysmal pricking or burning pain on the face, and a dislike of cold. The tongue coating is thin and white and the pulse efficient but rapid. Hyperactivity of the yang qi is present because of a deficiency of yin; the disease is of xu nature. It presents with an intermittent burning sensation on the face and irritability. The tongue coating is thin and yellow and the pulse bowstring and rapid.

Point Selection

1. Invasion of wind and cold

LI4 disperses wind.

SJ5 warms the middle jiao.

2. Hyperactivity of yang qi

St44 sedates the stomach

Liv3 tonifies the yin of the gan-liver.

Points may be selected according to the distribution of the trigeminal neuralgia: if the pain is particularly acute and severe select points on the painless side of the face.

Ophthalmic pain should be relieved by using local points, GB14, UB2 and Taiyang (Extra).

Maxillary pain should be treated by using SI18 and LI20.

Mandibular pain should be treated by using St4, St6 and St7.

Point Location

LI4.   In the middle of the first metacarpal on the radial aspect.

LI20.   Between the naso-labial groove and the mid-point of the outer border of the nasal ala.

St4.   On the corner of the mouth, directly below the middle of the eyebrow.

St6.   One finger's breadth anterior and superior to the lower angle of the mandible, where masseter attaches at the prominence of the muscle when the teeth are clenched.

St7.   In the depression of the lower border of the zygomatic arch, anterior to the condyloid process of the mandible.

St44.   Proximal to the web margin between the second and third toes in the depression distal and lateral to the second metatarso digital joint.

SI18.   Directly below the outer canthus of the eye in the depression below the lower border of the zygomatic bone.

Trigeminal Neuralgia

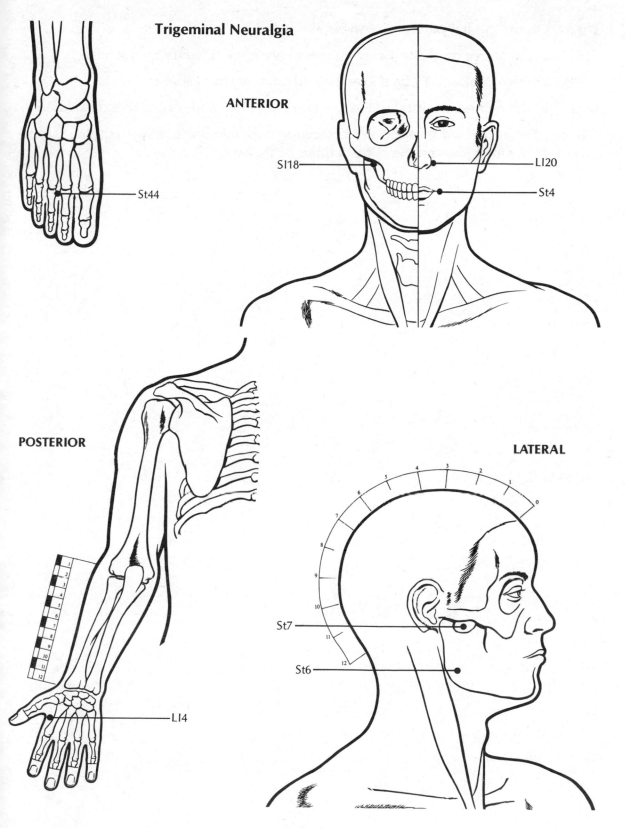

ANTERIOR

SI18

LI20

St4

St44

POSTERIOR

LI4

LATERAL

St7

St6

127

UB2.   On the medial extremity of the eyebrow.

SJ5.   2 cun above the posterior wrist crease between the radius and the ulna.

GB14. On the forehead, 1 cun above the mid-point of the eyebrow.

Liv3.   In the depression distal to the junction of the first and second metatarsal bones.

Taiyang (Extra). In the depression 1 cun posterior to the mid-point between the lateral end of the eyebrow and the outer canthus of the eye.

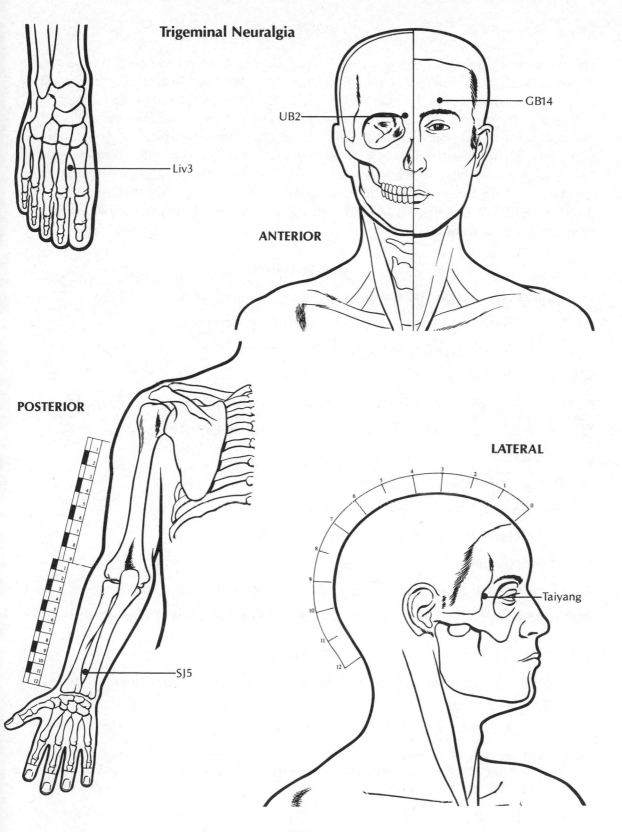

Trigeminal Neuralgia

Liv3

UB2

GB14

ANTERIOR

POSTERIOR

SJ5

LATERAL

Taiyang

VERTIGO

This is caused by a deficiency in the *pi-spleen* which results in the invasion of the pathogens *phlegm* and *damp*. These disturb the middle jiao and this in turn disturbs the mind resulting in vertigo. A weakness of the *shen-kidney* may also be associated with vertigo.

Invasion by *phlegm* and *damp* presents with dizziness, vertigo, blurred vision, lassitude and distension in the abdomen and chest. The tongue coating is white and greasy and the pulse soft and deficient. Deficiency of the *shen-kidney* (xu) presents with dizziness, blurred vision, a lumbar ache, pallor and weak lower extremities. The tongue proper is pale and tooth-marked, the tongue coating deficient and the pulse thready. If the *pi-spleen* is affected then it should be strengthened and the pathogens dispersed. If the *shen-kidney* is affected then it should be tonified.

Point Selection

1. Invasion by phlegm and damp

GB20. The Chinese name for this point is 'wind qi', and it is particularly useful for vertigo.

UB20 is the back shu point for tonifying the pi-spleen.

Sp6 tonifies the pi-spleen.

Ren12 strengthens the middle jiao, controlling the adverse ascent of qi to the head.

P6 stops the feeling of nausea and controls the adverse ascent of qi.

St40 disperses damp and phlegm.

2. Deficiency of the shen-kidney

K3 and K7 act together to tonify the shen-kidney.

UB23 is the back shu point representing the shen-kidney.

H7 pacifies the mind.

Ren4 is the point of general tonification and strengthens the body's resistance against disease.

GB20 and Ren12 should be used for the reasons stated above.

Point Location

St40.   8 cun superior and anterior to the lateral malleolus, two fingers' breadth lateral from the tibial crest.

Sp6.   3 cun above the medial malleolus just posterior to the tibial border.

H7.   On the transverse crease of the wrist in the articular region between the pisiform bone and the ulna, in the depression on the radial side of the tendon of flexor carpi ulnaris.

Vertigo

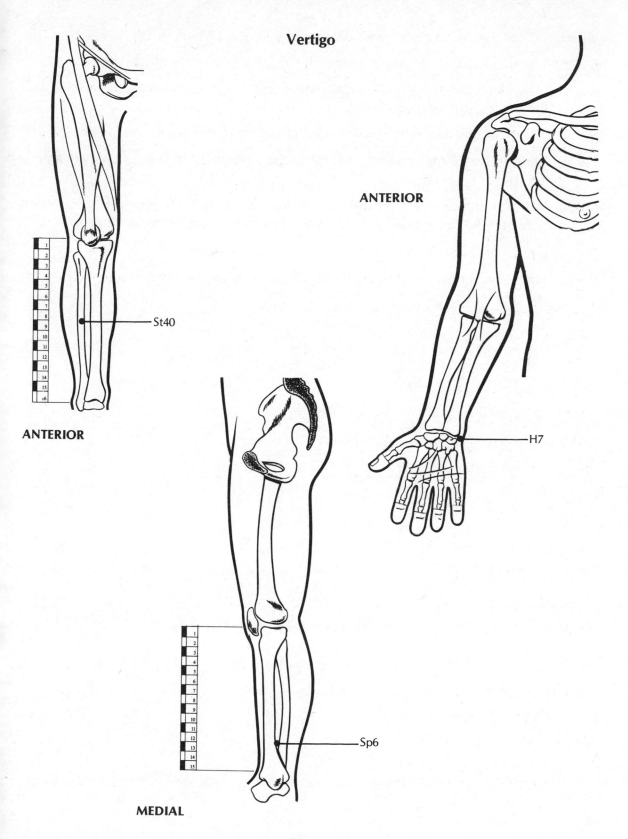

ANTERIOR

St40

ANTERIOR

H7

MEDIAL

Sp6

131

UB20. 1.5 cun lateral to the spinous process of T11.

UB23. 1.5 cun lateral to the lower border of the spinous process of L2.

K3. In the depression between the medial malleolus and the tendo-calcaneus, level with the tip of the medial malleolus.

K7. 2 cun directly above K3, on the anterior border of the tendo-calcaneus.

P6. 2 cun above the transverse crease to the wrist between the tendons of palmaris longus and flexor carpi radialis.

GB20. In the posterior aspect of the neck, below the occipital bone, in the depression between the upper portion of sternocleidomastoid and trapezius.

Ren4. On the mid-line of the abdomen 3 cun below the umbilicus.

Ren12. On the mid-line of the abdomen between the navel and the xiphisternum, 4 cun above the umbilicus.

Vertigo

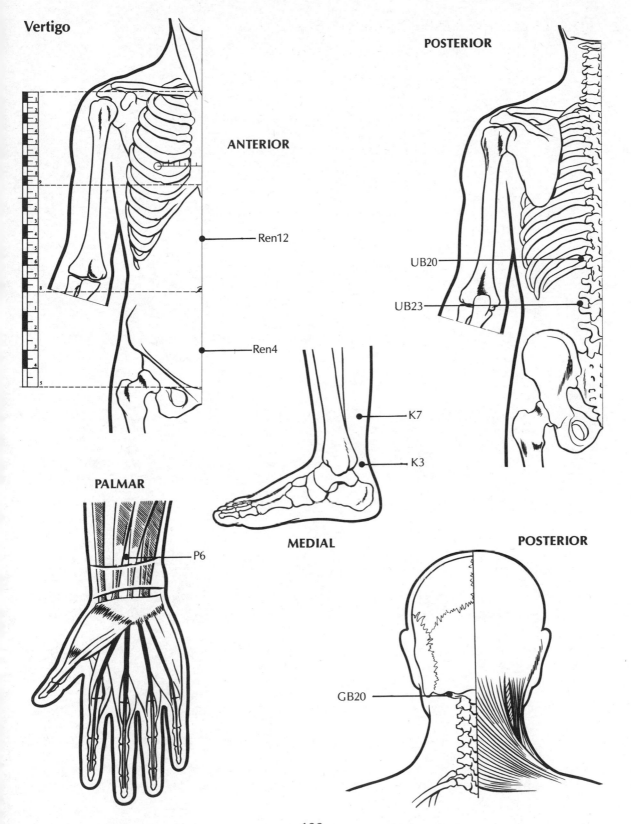

ANTERIOR

Ren12

Ren4

POSTERIOR

UB20

UB23

K7

K3

PALMAR

P6

MEDIAL

POSTERIOR

GB20

133

13.

Infectious Diseases

ACUTE RHINITIS (Coryza or the Common Cold)

The organ most commonly affected is the *fei-lung*. Deficiency of qi in the *fei-lung* allows the nose, its orifice, to be invaded by pathogens such as *wind, heat* and *cold*.

Invasion by *wind and cold* presents with severe nasal obstruction, a clear watery discharge and swollen nasal membranes. The tongue coating is white and the pulse deficient. Invasion by *wind and heat* presents with fever, headache and dark yellow urine. The tongue coating is yellow, the tongue proper red and the pulse large and rapid.

Therapy should be directed at clearing the pathogens (*wind, heat* and *cold*) and tonifying the *fei-lung*.

Point Selection

LI4 and LI11 disperse the pathogen wind.

LI4, LI11 and Du14 disperse the pathogen heat.

LI20 'frees' the nasal passages.

Lu7 tonifies and strengthens the qi of the fei-lung.

Yintang (Extra) should be used as a local point for headache. It also strengthens the function of Lu7.

Point Location

Lu7. Above the styloid process of the radius, 1.5 cun above the transverse wrist crease. Insert a one-inch needle obliquely towards the thumb.

LI4. In the middle of the first metacarpal on the radial aspect.

LI11. Midway between the lateral epicondyle and the lateral aspect of the cubital (elbow) crease, with the elbow flexed.

LI20. Between the naso-labial groove and the mid-point of the outer border of the nasal ala.

Du14. In the mid-line between the transverse process of C7 and T1.

Yintang (Extra). Midway between the medial end of the two eyebrows (the glabella).

Acute Rhinitis

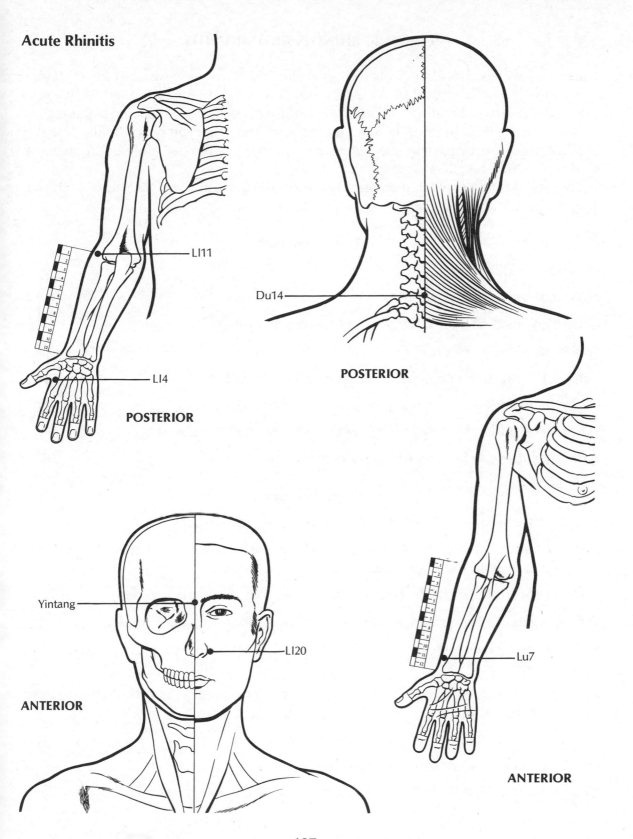

LI11

Du14

LI4

POSTERIOR

POSTERIOR

Yintang

LI20

ANTERIOR

Lu7

ANTERIOR

137

CHRONIC RHINITIS AND SINUSITIS

This occurs if there is deficiency of *fei-lung* causing an accumulation of pathogenic factors. Occasionally a deficiency of qi in the *pi-spleen* may affect the *large intestine* and weaken the *fei-lung* (the large intestine and lung are linked) predisposing to the invasion of pathogens.

Wind and *cold* are the most common pathogens. The tongue proper is usually pale and tooth-marked, the tongue coating is greasy if the pi-spleen is affected and white if excessive cold is present. The pulse is deficient.

Therapy should be directed at dispersing the pathogens and tonifying the qi of the fei-lung and/or pi-spleen.

Point Selection

LI4 and LI11 disperse wind.

LI20 frees the nasal passages.

UB13 and UB43 free the flow of qi and tonify the fei-lung.

Sp6 tonifies the pi-spleen.

Yintang (Extra) strengthens the function of UB13 and UB43.

UB2 can be added to alleviate pain caused by frontal sinusitis.

SI18 can be added to alleviate the pain caused by maxillary sinusitis.

Taiyang (Extra) can be used for the symptom headache.

Point Location

LI4. In the middle of the first metacarpal on the radial aspect.

LI11. Midway between the lateral epicondyle and the lateral aspect of the cubital (elbow) crease, with the elbow flexed.

LI20. Between the naso-labial groove and the mid-point of the outer border of the nasal ala.

Sp6. 3 cun above the medial malleolus just posterior to the tibial border.

SI18. Directly below the outer canthus in the depression below the lower border of the zygomatic bone.

UB2. In the depression proximal to the medial end of the eyebrow directly above the inner canthus of the eye.

UB13. 1.5 cun lateral to the spinous process of T3.

UB43. 3 cun lateral to the spinous process of T4.

Yintang (Extra). Midway between the medial end of the two eyebrows (the glabella).

Chronic Rhinitis and Sinusitis

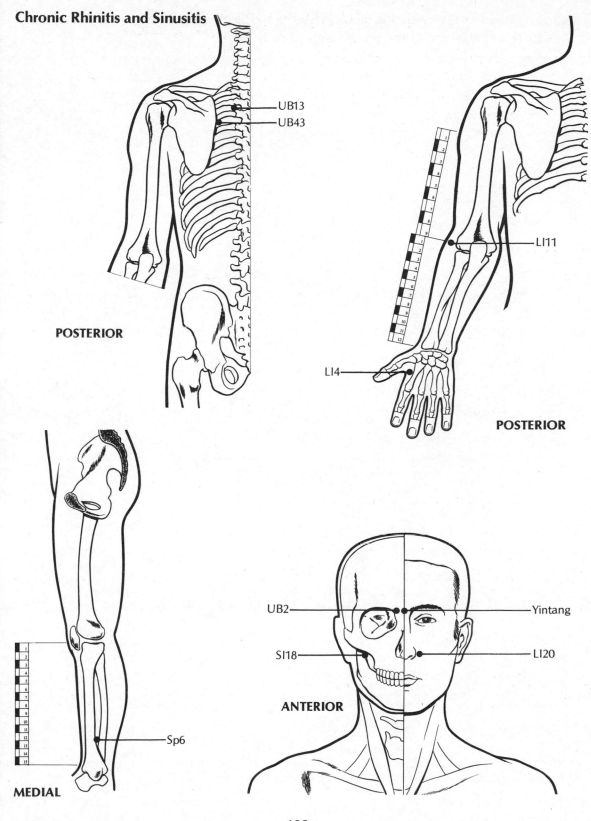

POSTERIOR

UB13
UB43

POSTERIOR

LI11

LI4

MEDIAL

Sp6

ANTERIOR

UB2

SI18

Yintang

LI20

Taiyang (Extra). In the depression 1 cun posterior to the mid-point between the lateral end of the eyebrow and the outer canthus of the eye.

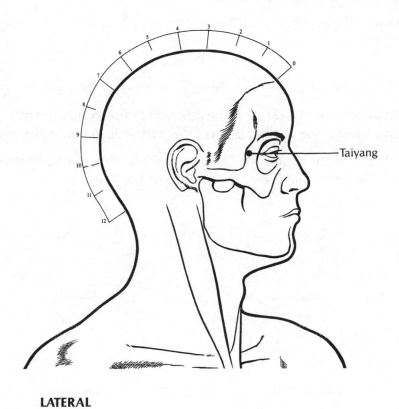

Taiyang

LATERAL

CONJUNCTIVITIS

This is caused by *wind and heat* invading the eye resulting in a red, painful purulent eye. The treatment is to clear *wind* and *heat* on a symptomatic basis.

Point Selection

LI4 removes heat and inflammation.

Taiyang (Extra) removes local heat.

GB41 sedates the gan-liver and is symptomatically successful in resolving conjunctivitis.

Point Location

LI4.   In the middle of the first metacarpal on the radial aspect.

GB41. In the depression distal to the junction of the fourth and fifth metatarsal bones on the lateral side of the tendon of extensor digiti minimi of the foot.

Taiyang (Extra). In the depression 1 cun posterior to the mid-point between the lateral end of the eyebrow and the outer canthus of the eye.

Conjunctivitis

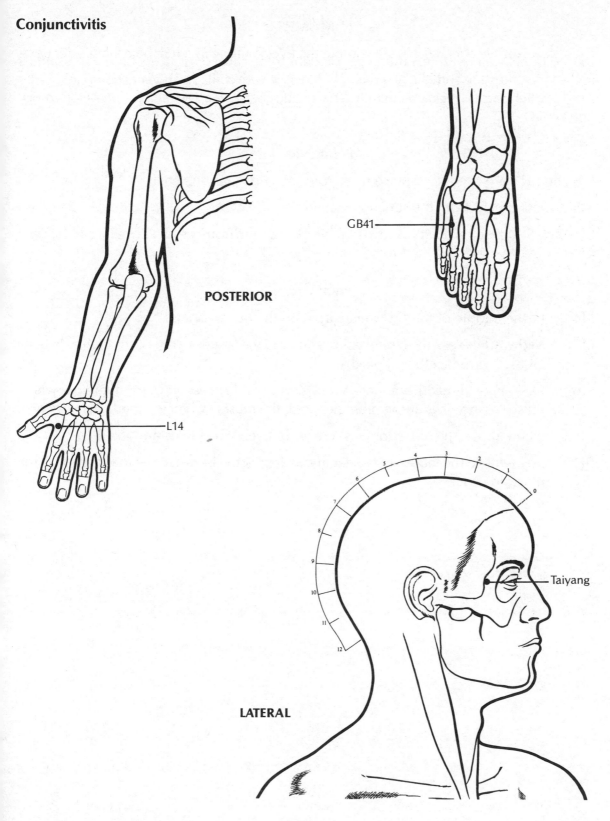

POSTERIOR

GB41

L14

Taiyang

LATERAL

143

MUMPS

In traditional Chinese terms mumps is thought to be caused by an accumulation of *heat* in the large intestine and sanjiao channels. It begins with chills and fever accompanied with a red swollen parotid region bilaterally. The tongue coating is greasy and the pulse superficial and rapid.

Point Selection

LI4 and LI11 are used to disperse heat from the large intestine channel.

SJ5 disperses heat from the sanjiao channel.

SJ17 and St6 are local points used to remove obstruction from the local swelling and relieve pain.

Point Location

LI4.   In the middle of the first metacarpal on the radial aspect.

LI11.   Midway between the lateral epicondyle and the lateral aspect of the cubital (elbow) crease, with the elbow flexed.

St6.   One finger's breadth anterior and superior to the lower angle of the mandible, where masseter attaches at the prominence of the muscle when the teeth are clenched.

SJ5.   2 cun above the posterior wrist crease between the radius and the ulna.

SJ17.   Posterior to the lobule of the ear in the depression between the mandible and the mastoid process.

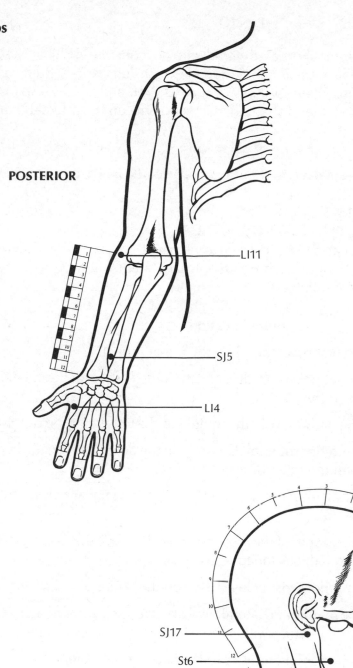

POSTERIOR

LI11

SJ5

LI4

SJ17

St6

LATERAL

POLIO

The sequelae of polio are commonly treated with electro-acupuncture in China. The Chinese believe that malnourishment of the tendons, due to exhaustion of body fluid caused by invasion of the *fei-lung* by exogenous pathogens such as *wind* and *heat,* is responsible for polio. The treatment is to tonify and strengthen lower points on the affected limbs.

Point Selection

The following points can be selected for treatment of affected limbs; they should be used only on the affected side.

1. Upper limb, LI4, LI11, LI15, SJ5.
2. Lower limb, St31, St36, St41, GB30, GB34, GB39.

These points should be stimulated electrically on a number of occasions; use high frequency stimulation for at least an hour at each treatment. Treatment will need to be repeated frequently if results are to be obtained.

Point Location

LI4.   In the middle of the first metacarpal on the radial aspect.

LI11.   Midway between the lateral epicondyle and the lateral aspect of the cubital (elbow) crease, with the elbow flexed.

LI15.   Antero inferior to the acromion, in the middle of the upper portion of the deltoid.

St31.   Directly below the anterior superior iliac spine in the depression on the lateral side of the sartorius, when the thigh is flexed.

St36.   3 cun below the lateral aspect of the knee joint line, one finger's breadth from the anterior crest of the tibia.

St41.   At the junction of the dorsum of the foot and the leg between the tendons of extensor digitorum longus and hallicus longus.

SJ5.   2 cun above the posterior wrist crease between the radius and the ulna.

GB30.   At the junction of the middle and lateral third of a line joining the greater trochanter and the sacral hiatus; puncture with a three-inch needle deep into the pyriformis.

GB34.   In the depression anterior and inferior to the head of the fibula.

GB39.   3 cun above the tip of the lateral malleolus in the depression between the posterior border of the fibula and the tendons of peroneus longus and brevis.

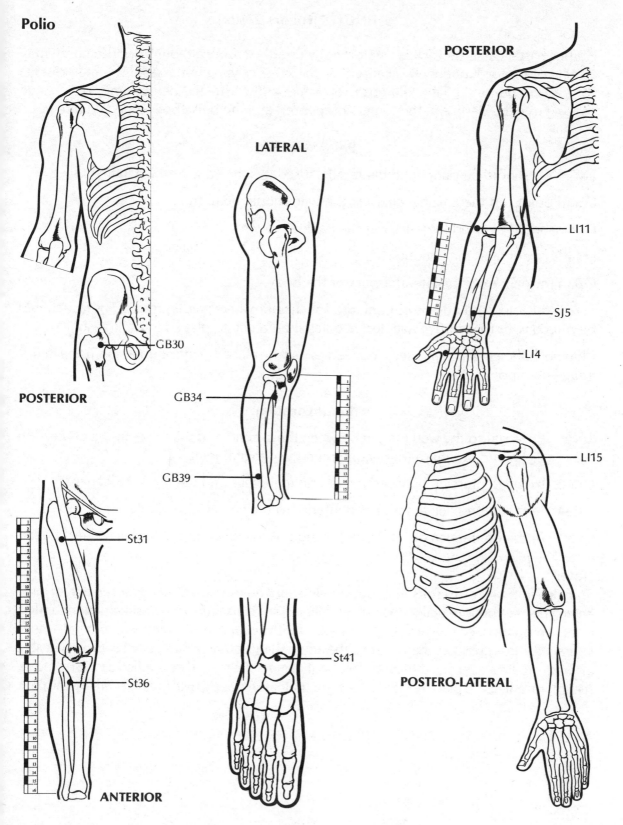

Polio

POSTERIOR

GB30

POSTERIOR

St31

St36

ANTERIOR

LATERAL

GB34

GB39

St41

POSTERIOR

LI11

SJ5

LI4

LI15

POSTERO-LATERAL

147

SHINGLES (Herpes Zoster)

Herpes zoster can affect any dermatome, it is usually sensory although occasionally it may affect the motor function. It is caused by an excess of yang of the *gan-liver* and presents with severe burning pain and a pustular rash over the affected dermatome. The tongue coating may be deficient, the tongue proper red and the pulse bowstring and thready.

Point Selection

Liv3. This should be punctured bilaterally, it sedates the yang of the gan-liver.

Distal points on the channel crossing the pain should be used.

UB60 should be used for pain over the back.

St44 for pain over the abdomen.

GB34 for pain over the lateral aspect of the body.

The distal points should only be punctured on the side where pain is present. The rash should be ringed with four or five needles, needles should *not* be placed into the rash.

Channel balancing may be used, i.e., needles may be placed in the normal side, using mirror image pain points.

Point Location

St44.   Proximal to the web margin between the second and third toes in the depression distal and lateral to the second metatarso digital joint.

UB60.   In the depression between the lateral malleolus and the tendo-calcaneus.

GB34.   In the depression anterior and inferior to the head of the fibula.

Liv3.   In the depression distal to the junction of the first and second metatarsal bones.

Note:

Shingles in the West results in about one in every hundred patients over the age of sixty having post-herpetic neuralgia (pain after shingles). In China little or no post-herpetic neuralgia is seen, probably because all shingles is treated with acupuncture. *Treatment of post-herpetic neuralgia* is less effective than treating the acute shingles (nerve damage may be irreversible after the acute stage), but the same therapeutic principles should be applied as with shingles. It is important not to place needles into the neuralgic area as this will only exacerbate the pain.

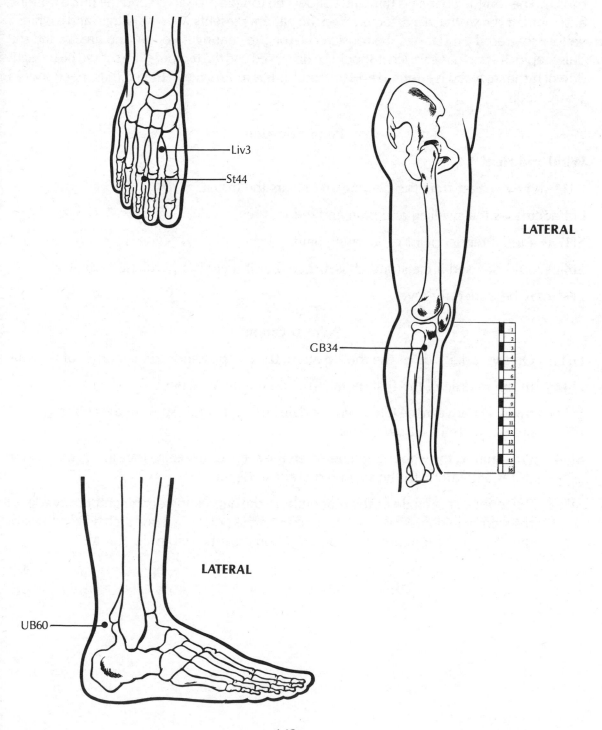

TONSILLITIS

This is due to invasion by *wind and heat*. The *stomach* is frequently affected by this. If *wind* and *heat* invade then the tonsillitis is of abrupt onset and associated with fever and red swollen tonsils. The tongue coating is thin and yellow, the tongue proper red and the pulse floating and rapid. If the *stomach* is affected then the patient presents with dysphagia and a whitish yellow scattered exudate on the tonsils. The tongue coating is yellow and greasy and the pulse rapid. If *wind* has invaded it should be dispersed and the temperature should be brought down. If the *stomach* is affected and the tonsillitis is more severe, then the stomach should be treated.

Point Selection

Wind and Heat

Lu11 removes heat from the fei-lung and clears the throat.

LI4 decreases the swelling and pain and reduces fever.

SI17 is a local tender point for treating pain.

St44 should be used if the stomach is affected or if there is a purulent tonsillitis.

LI11 may be added for fever.

Point Location

Lu11. On the radial side of the thumb about 0.1 cun posterior to the corner of the nail.

LI4. In the middle of the first metacarpal on the radial aspect.

LI11. Midway between the lateral epicondyle and the lateral aspect of the cubital (elbow) crease, with the elbow flexed.

St44. Proximal to the web margin between the second and third toes in the depression distal and lateral to the second metatarso digital joint.

SI17. Posterior to the angle of the mandible, in the depression on the anterior border of the sternocleidomastoid. When puncturing this point use a one-inch needle towards the root of the tongue, needling sensation must be felt in the throat.

Tonsillitis

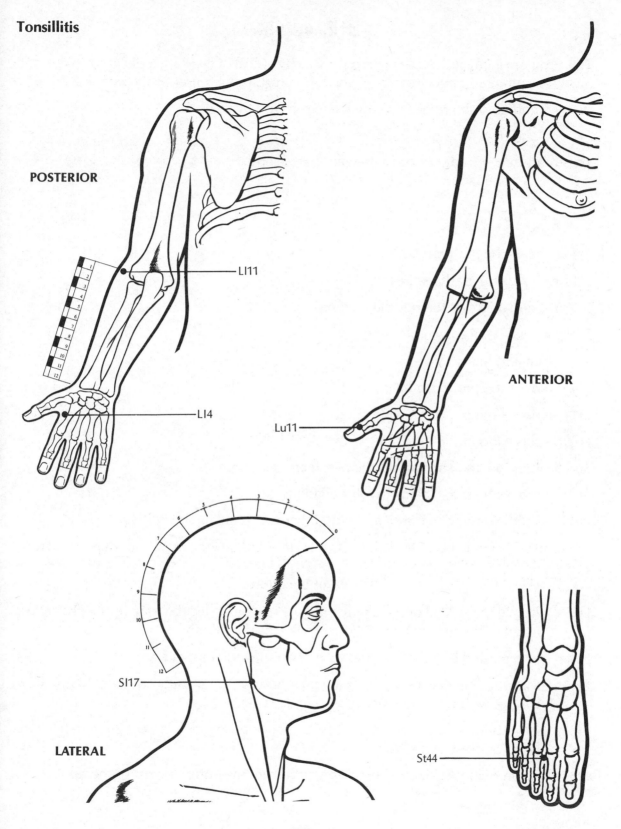

POSTERIOR

LI11

LI4

ANTERIOR

Lu11

LATERAL

SI17

St44

151

URTICARIA (Hives)

This problem is caused by the invasion of *wind* and *heat* or *wind* and *cold* into the skin and muscles. Impaired circulation of qi and blood results, the onset of the rash is abrupt.

In wind and cold the rash is pale pink and relieved by warmth.

In wind and heat the rash is red, hot and itchy.

The treatment is to disperse the relevant pathogens.

Point Selection

1. Wind and cold

LI4 removes the pathogen wind.

LI11 removes the pathogen wind.

Lu7 dispels wind and tonifies the fei-lung.

Sp6 tonifies the pi-spleen.

2. Wind and heat

LI4 removes the pathogen heat.

LI11 removes the pathogen wind.

Lu7 dispels wind and tonifies the fei-lung.

Sp6 tonifies yin and strengthens the pi-spleen.

Sp10 removes heat and helps to relieve itching.

UB17 aids the circulation of qi and blood thereby resolving the itching.

St36 and St37 should be added if there is gastro-intestinal involvement and/or epigastric pain.

Point Location

Lu7.   Above the styloid process of the radius, 1.5 cun above the transverse wrist crease. Insert a one-inch needle obliquely towards the thumb.

LI4.   In the middle of the first metacarpal on the radial aspect.

LI11.   Midway between the lateral epicondyle and the lateral aspect of the cubital (elbow) crease, with the elbow flexed.

St36.   3 cun below the lateral aspect of the knee joint line, one finger's breadth from the anterior crest of the tibia.

St37.   3 cun below St36, one finger's breadth from the anterior crest of the tibia.

Urticaria

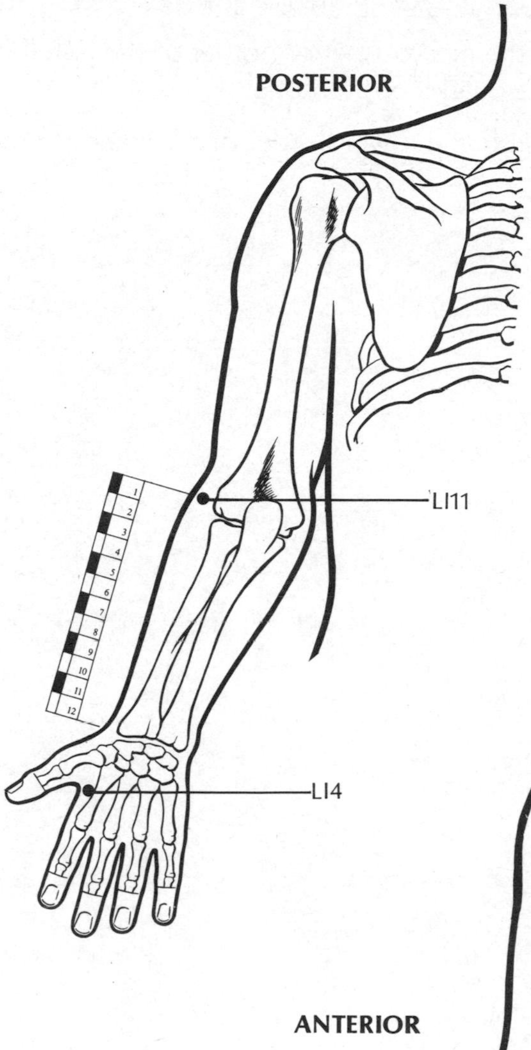

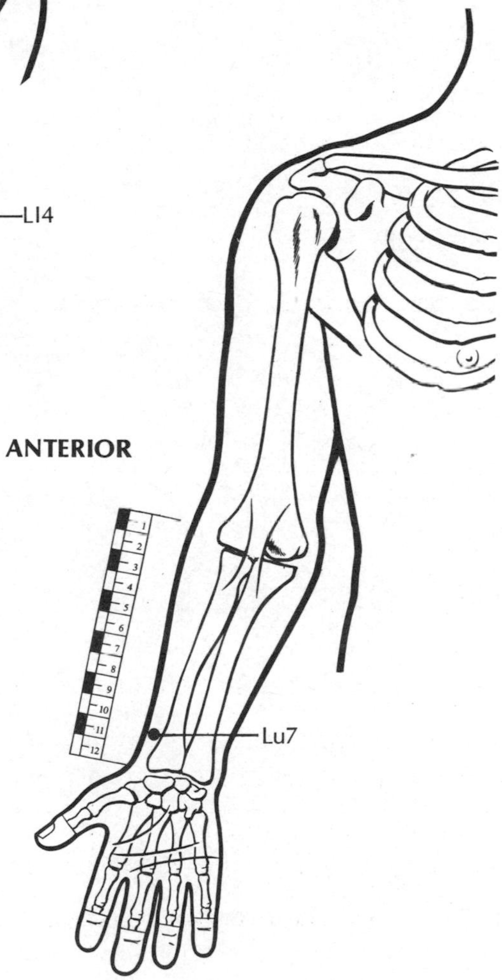

POSTERIOR

LI11

LI4

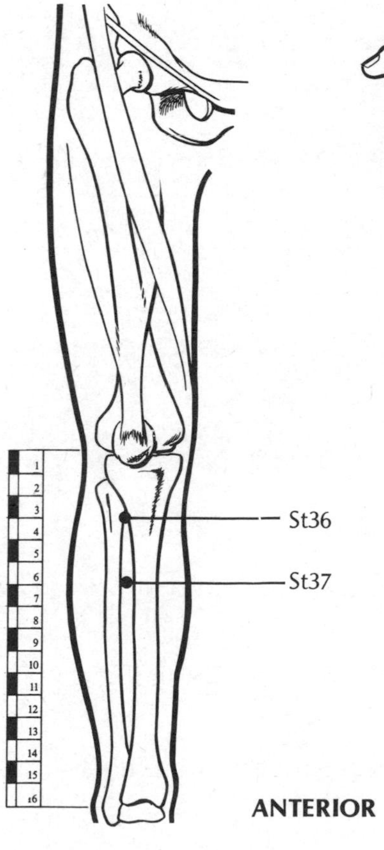

ANTERIOR

St36

St37

ANTERIOR

Lu7

Sp6. 3 cun above the medial malleolus just posterior to the tibial border.

Sp10. 2 cun above the mediosuperior border of the patella on the bulge of the medial portion of the quadriceps femoris.

UB17. 1.5 cun lateral to the lower border of the spinous process of T7.

Urticaria (Hives)

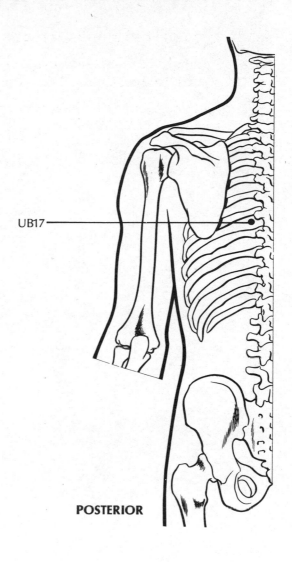

UB17

POSTERIOR

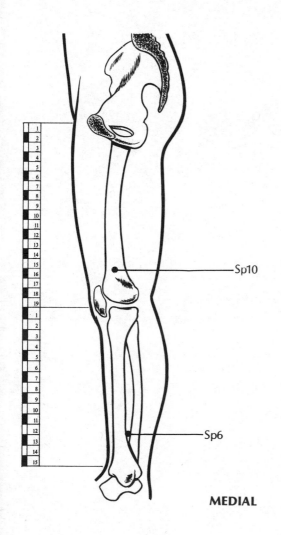

Sp10

Sp6

MEDIAL

References

Introduction

1. Ding, Roath and Lewith, *American Journal of Acupuncture,* Volume 11, 1983, 51-54.

2. Ma, et al, 'National Symposium of Acupuncture and Moxibustion and Acupuncture Anaesthesia', Peking, 1979, 513.

3. Zang Fachu, et al, 'National Symposium of Acupuncture and Moxibustion and Acupuncture Anaesthesia', Peking, 1979, 8.

4. Tang Zhaoling, et al, 'National Symposium of Acupuncture and Moxibustion and Acupuncture Anaesthesia', Peking, 1979, 51.

5. Anon, *Journal of Chinese Medicine,* Volume II, 1974, 216.

6. Anon, *Chinese Medical Journal,* Volume 1, 1975, 247.

7. O'Connor and Bensky, *American Journal of Chinese Medicine,* Volume 3, 1975, 377.

8. Dai, et al, *American Journal of Chinese Medicine,* Volume 2, 1974, 181.

Index

Essentials of Chinese Acupuncture, 28